DAILY VAGUS NERVE EXERCISES

Self-Help Exercises to Stimulate Vagal Tone. Relieve Anxiety, Prevent Inflammation, Reduce Chronic Illness, Anxiety, Depression, Trauma, PTSD and Lots More

Marcus Porges

TABLES OF CONTENTS

INTRODUCTION

What is the vagus nerve and why is it so important?

Simply put, the vagus nerve is the commander-in-chief of your inner nerve center, regulating all of your major organs. This is the longest cranial nerve, which starts in the brain just behind the ears and connects to all the body's major organs. It sends fibers from your brain-stem to all of your visceral organs, and is literally the commander of your inner nerve center, communicating nerve impulses to every organ in your body. The word vagus literally means "wanderer", because it wanders throughout the body from the brain all the way to the fertility organs, hitting everything in between. When it comes to mind-body connection, the vagus nerve is monumental, since it reaches all the major organs except for the adrenal and thyroid glands.

This is an important nerve to every organ it is in contact with. It is what helps control anxiety and depression in the brain. How we connect with one another is closely related to the vagus nerve as its attached to nerves that tune our ears to speech, it coordinates eye contact, and those which regulate expressions. This nerve also has the power to affect proper hormone release in the body which keeps our mental and physical systems healthy.

It is the vagus nerve that is responsible for increasing stomach acidity and digestive juice secretion for ease in digestion in the stomach. When stimulated, it can also help you to absorb vitamin B12. When it is not working properly, you can then expect to have serious gut issues such as Colitis, IBS, and Re-flux, just to name a few. Reflux issues are due to a vagus nerve issue because the it also controls the esophagus. It's the improper reflex of the esophagus that causes conditions like Gerd and Reflux.

The vagus nerve also helps control the heart rate and blood pressure, preventing heart disease. While in the liver and pancreas, it's this nerve that controls blood glucose balance, preventing diabetes. When it passes through the gallbladder, the vagus nerve helps to release bile, which is what assists your body in eliminating toxins and breaking down fat. While in the bladder, it's this nerve that promotes general kidney function, increasing blood flow, thereby improving filtration in our bodies. When the vagus nerve gets to the spleen, activation will reduce inflammation in all target organs. This nerve even has the power to control fertility and orgasms in women. An inactive or blocked vagus nerve can wreak havoc throughout the mind and body.

Now that we know that the vagus nerve is connected to all the major organs and proper functioning of those organs, we can easily conclude that any disorder, illness, or disease of the mind, body, or spirit, can be reversed or even cured by activating and stimulating the vagus nerve. So you will indeed see positive effects from vagus nerve stimulation on issues such as anxiety disorders, heart disease, headaches and migraines, fibromyalgia, alcohol addiction, circulation, gut issues, memory issues, mood disorders, MS, and even cancer.

There are many documented ways to stimulate the vagus nerve such as singing or chanting, laughter, yoga, meditation, breathing exercises, exercise in general, and sound just to name a few. Singing and laughter works the muscles at the back of your throat which activates the nerve. Mild exercising and exercising in general increases gut fluids which means that the vagus nerve has been stimulated. A regimented Yoga practice can also increase activation of this nerve due to the movements but also the Meditation and OMing helps stimulate the vagus nerve. All of these ways you can use stimulate the vagus nerve have one thing in common: Sound!!

Findings of resonant frequency of organs is happening worldwide by doctors to aid in vibrating the body back into a state of health, and transfuses illness and diseases such as anxiety, PTSD, migraines, depression, memory issues, chronic pain, sleep disorders, and even cancer. "You can really look at disease as a form or disharmony," says Dr. Gaynor director of oncology at the Strang-Cornell Cancer Prevention Center in New York, and author of Sounds of Healing. "We know that sound and music have profound effects on the immune system, which clearly do have a lot to do with cancer."

There was also a study in April of 2016, that involved patient with Alzheimer's Disease. Researchers from the University of Toronto, Wilfrid Laurier University, and the Baycrest Centre Hospitals conducted a study of these patients in different stages of the disease, subjecting them to sound simulation at 40 hertz. They noted "promising" results with cognition, clarity, and alertness. Lee Bartel, one of the authors of these findings stated that, "Parts of the brain appear to be at the same communication frequency, and that frequency is about 40 Hz. So when you have a deterioration of that when you have too little of it the two parts of the brain that want to talk to each other, like the thalamus and the hippo campus, the short term memory to the long-term memory, they can't talk to each other, they won't communicate, so you won't have long-term memory." Bartel explained that the sound-simulation treatment at 40 Hz leads to an "increased" frequency, which allows "parts of the brain to talk to each other again."

One specific school of thought comes from a French otolaryngologist, Alfred A Tomatis, who believes that the primary function of the ear is to provide all the cells of the body with electrical stimulation, thereby "toning up the whole system and imparting greater dynamism to the human being" (Tomatis. 1978) He believes that sounds abundant in high harmonics are considered charging sounds, and sounds abundant in lower tones are considered to be discharging sounds. Tomatis claimed to have successfully treated a wide variety of illness through sound because they were all related to issues with the inner ear. Just a few of the issues he's successfully treated were stuttering, depression, ADD, concentration issues, and disorders related to balance.

There is another study that suggests that the Tomatis Method is supportive to assisting children with ADD. "Results revealed statistically significant improvements for the Tomatis when compared to the nonTomatis group: the experimental group showed the significant improvements in processing speed, phonological awareness, phonemic decoding efficiency when reading, behavior, and auditory attention."

Sound is rapidly becoming one of the most largely buzzed about gatekeepers of health in alternative healing modalities today! Sound is a brilliant implementation of common medicine to stimulate the vagus nerve promoting the health and vitality of all the organs in your body. Do this through sound healing and Crystal Chakra Singing Bowls. Clear Quartz is called the 'Master Healer' because is has the ability to amplify, transform, and transfer energy. When working with these quartz crystal bowls, the effects on the organs, tissues, and cells, along with the circulatory, endocrine, and metabolic systems are intense. The tones from the crystals are heard by the ear, felt in the body, stimulate the vagus nerve, enabling the vibrations to echo also through each Chakra center in the body, creating a balanced and rejuvenated mind, body & spirit!

Vagus Nerve Stimulation - Control Epilepsy

Quantum Brain Healing relies on a base of orthomolecular medicine including aminoacids, vitamins, minerals, herbs, botanical extracts, Chinese herbal formulas, and many alternative therapies. There is no answer that will address healing for everyone. It is always key to remain open to technology when other options have not met our goals. One option that can be looked after trying nutritional therapy is Vagus Nerve Stimulation. This is a medical device that is surgically implanted. Any major medical center in the US and Europe can implant this device for a patient that qualifies.

Vagus Nerve Stimulation (VNS) involves sending a message to the brain using periodic mild electrical stimulation from the vagus nerve in the neck by a surgically implanted small medical device. There is no brain surgery involved. This stimulation or pulse is sent by a medical device similar to a pacemaker. The vagus nerve is part of the autonomic nervous system and controls involuntary body functions.

VNS may control epilepsy in cases where antiepileptic drugs are ineffective or have intolerable side effects, or neurosurgery is not appropriate for some reason. VNS is effective in stopping seizures in some patients.

The implanted medical device is a flat, round battery, and measures about the size of a silver dollar. The VNS medical device was developed by Cyberonics, Inc. The doctor determines the strength and timing of the pulses administered by the device according to each patient's individual needs. The level of electrical stimulation can be changed without additional surgery with a programming wand connected to a laptop computer.

The side effects of VNS during treatment may include hoarseness, coughing, throat pain, shortness of breath, a short and slight sensation of choking, altered voice sound, ear pain, tooth pain, and a tingling sensation in the neck. Skin irritation or infection could occur at the implantation site. VNS does not negatively impact the brain. This is major surgery and should not be considered lightly. For those with uncontrollable epileptic seizures, it may be last option. Consider all options before giving up on controlling seizure. This is not neurosurgery and it is safer.

Dealing with Anxiety Using your Vagus Nerve

How often do you have to deal with anxiety in your everyday life?

If you find yourself worrying too much or getting caught into non-stopping irrational thoughts or even feeling nausea, chest pain and heart palpitations then this book is for you.

You are about to learn a simple yet very effective technique to deal with anxiety naturally by stimulating your vagus nerve. This powerful technique can be used to relieve stress and anxiety anywhere and anytime; at home, when commuting and of course at those horrible work meetings.

Did you know that the FDA approved a surgically implanted device that is successfully treating depression by periodically stimulating the vagus nerve?

But hopefully you won't need surgery. You can enjoy the benefits of vagus nerve stimulation by adopting some simple breathing techniques.

So what is that vagus nerve?

The vagus nerve is the most important element of the parasympathetic nervous system (the one that calms you down by controlling your relaxation response).

It originates from the brainstem and it is "wandering" all the way down, into the belly, spreading fibers to the tongue, pharynx, vocal chords, lungs, heart, stomach, intestines and glands that produce antistress enzymes and hormones (like Acetylcholine, Prolactin, Vasopressin, Oxytocin), influencing digestion, metabolism and of course the relaxation response.

Vagus nerve acts as the mind-body connection, and it is the cabling behind your heart's emotions and gut instincts. The key to manage your mind state and your anxiety levels lies on being able to activate the calming nervous pathways of your parasympathetic system.

You cannot control this part of the nervous system on demand, but you can indirectly stimulate your vagus nerve by:

Immersing your face in cold water (diving reflex)

Attempting to exhale against a closed airway (Valsalva maneuver).

This can be done by keeping the mouth closed and pinching the nose while trying to breathe out. This greatly increases pressures inside the chest cavity stimulating the vagus nerve and increasing vagal tone

Singing

And of course, diaphragmatic breathing techniques

Strengthening this living nervous system can pay great dividends, and the best tool to achieve that is by training your breath.

Breathe with your diaphragm

Now it's time to put this concept into practice. The first thing you need to do is breathe using your diaphragm (abdominal breathing). This is the foundation of proper breathing and anxiety relief.

The diaphragm is your primary breathing muscle. It is belled shaped and when you inhale it patterns out (or should flatten out), acting as piston and creating vacuum on you thoracic cavity, so your lungs can expand and air gets in.

On the other side it creates pressure, pushing the viscera down and out, expanding your belly. That's why good breathing practice is described as abdominal breathing or belly breathing.

Breathe with the glottis partially closed

Glottis is at the back of your tongue and it is closed when you are holding your breath. Here we want have it partially closed. It is that feeling you have in your throat while you exhale and make a "Hhhhh" sound in order to clean your glasses, but without actually making the sound.

16

It also resembles the way you breathe when you are in the verge of sleep and you are about to snore a little bit.

By controlling the glottis you are:

Controlling the air flow, both during inhale and during exhale

Stimulating your vagus nerve.

Try it right now

Now it's time to put all this theory into action by practicing this 7 - 11 diaphragmatic breathing technique.

Inhale diaphragmatically through your nose, with your glottis partially closed, like almost making a "Hhhhh" sound for a count of 7

Hold your breath for a moment

Exhale through your nose (or you mouth), with your glottis partially closed, like almost making a "Hhhhh" sound for a count of 11

This is one breath cycle; go for 6 - 12 cycles and observe the results.

Practice, Practice, Practice

The more you practice the more effective this technique will be.

Eventually, when your newly acquired breathing skill is established and abdominal breathing becomes a habit, you'll find your body constantly operating at a much lower stress level.

You will also notice (or sometimes you will not even notice it) how your breath responses to stressful situations; your body will be conditioned to automatically control your breath and by this, your stress and anxiety.

Vagus Nerve Stimulation Therapy Helps Eliminate Drug Cravings, Finds Study

Addiction to any substance can make the life of an individual topsy-turvy. From spending a fortune to deceiving own family, a person addicted to illegal substances can go to any extent. But how does addiction force someone to put so much at stake and then lose all? There are several factors at play when it comes to dealing with the growing problem of addiction.

Cravings are a serious issue that torment numerous people fighting drug addiction, especially when they try to come off the addictive substance. Ironically, many people would have successfully attained long-term sobriety if cravings did not crop up with addiction. Apart from being considered as the major obstacles in recovery treatment, cravings are also the root cause of relapse.

A complete recovery from addiction happens only when a person is free from cravings. Living a drug-free life without the need for constant monitoring against drug cravings can be difficult for a recovering individual, but a recent study published in the journal Learning and Memory has suggested that drug cravings can be effectively treated with vagus nerve stimulation (VNS) therapy. Under the therapy, the patients are taught new behaviors that replace their old addictive behavior of seeking drugs.

Role of VNS in addiction recovery

In the University of Texas at Dallas study, the researchers revealed that the VNS therapy helped patients to recover from the maladaptive behavior of drug taking. VNS is basically a surgical process wherein a device is implanted to a wire threaded along the vagus nerve, which travels up from the neck to the brain and connects with the area responsible for regulating mood. Sized as small as a silver dollar, the device works just like a pacemaker. It primarily works by sending a slight electric pulses through the vagus nerve, which further reaches to the brain, thereby controlling the cravings and urges.

The methodology is approved by the U.S. Food and Drug Administration (FDA) and is considered as a potential treatment for treatment-resistant depression, post-traumatic stress disorder (PTSD) and paralysis. The study further highlighted that VNS facilitates "extinction learning" of drugseeking behaviors by reducing cravings and replacing the behavior associated with addiction with new ones. "Extinction of fearful memories and extinction of drugseeking memories relies on the same substrate in the brain. In our experiments, VNS facilitates both the extinction learning and reduces the relapse response as well," said Dr. Sven Kroener of the University of Texas at Dallas.

Drug-free life is possible

Though addictive substances succeed in temporarily alleviating emotional and physical pains of drug abusers, they have to eventually cope with the painful symptoms of substance abuse. Besides developing a number of physical and mental problems, many of these individuals also become self destructive and suicidal in nature.

Addiction to any substance can be life threatening. Only a comprehensive treatment program involving detoxification, medications, psychotherapies and other experiential therapies like yoga, meditation etc. can help an individual get sober. Moreover, a holistic recovery management plan is equally important to sustain the period of sobriety and manage cravings. However, the extent to which health care practitioners can garner results in the treatment for drug addiction is dependent on the clinical characteristics of the patients that may vary according to the type of drug being abused as well as its quantity, duration and the method of using the drug (oral or intravenous).

The Glossopharyngeal Nerve and Vagus Nerve (Cranial Nerves IX and X) and Their Disorders

Since these two cranial nerves are intimately connected, they are described here together. The glossopharyngeal nerve has a sensory and motor component. The motor fibers arise from the nucleus ambiguous situated in the lateral part of the medulla. Along with the vagus and accessory nerves, they leave the skull through the jugular foramen. They supply the stylopharyngeus muscle whose function is to elevate the pharynx. Autonomic efferent fibers of the glossopharyngeal nerve arise from the inferior salivatory nucleus. The preganglionic fibers pass to the otic ganglion through the lesser superficial petrosal nerve. and postganglionic fibers pass through the auriculotemporal branch of the fifth nerve to reach to reach the Parotid gland. The nuclei of the sensory fibers of the glossopharyngeal nerve are situated in the petrous ganglion which lies within the petrous bone below the jugular foramen and also the superior ganglion, which is small. The exteroceptive fibers supply the faucial tonsils, posterior wall of the pharynx, part of the soft palate and taste sensations from the posterior third of the tongue.

The vagus: This is the longest among all the cranial nerves. The motor fibers arise from the nucleu ambiguus and supply all the muscles of the pharynx, soft palate and larynx, with the exception of tensor veli palati and stylopharyngeus. The parasympathetic fibers arise from the dorsal efferent nucleus and leave the medulla as preganglionic fibers of the craniosacral portion of the autonomic nervous system. These fibers terminate on ganglia close to the viscera which they supply by post-ganglionic fibers. The are parasympatahetic in function. Thus vagal stimulation produces bradycardia, bronchial constriction, secretion of gastric and pancreatic juice and increased peristalsis. The sensory portion of the vagus has its nuclei in the jugular in ganglion and ganglion nodosum. The vagus carries sensations from the posterior aspect of the external auditory meatus and adjacent pinna and pain sensation from the duramater lining the posterior cranial fossa.

Testing: It is better to test the 9th and 10th nerve functions together as they are affected usually together. Inquire for symptoms like dysphagia, dysarthria, nasal regurgitation of fluids and hoarseness of voice. The motor part is tested by examining the uvula when the patient is made to open his mouth. The Uvula is normally in the midline. In unilateral vagal paralysis, the palatal arch is flattened and lowered ipsilaterally. On phonation, the uvula is deviated to the normal side.

The gag reflex or the pharyngeal reflex is elicited by applying a stimulus, such as a tongue balde or cotton to the psoterior pharyngeal wall or tonsillar region. If the reflex is present, there will be elevation and contraction of the pharyngeal musculature accompanied by retraction of the tongue. The afferent arch of this

23

reflex is subserved by the glossopharyngeal while the efferent is through the vagus. This reflex is lost in either 9th or 10th nerve lesions. Test for general sensations over the posterior pharyngeal wall, soft palate and faucial tonsils, and taste over the posterior third of the tongue. These are impaired in glossopharyngeal paralysis.

Disorders of ninth and tenth nerve functions

Isolated involvement of either nerve is rare and usually they are involved together, often the eleventh and twelfth nerves may also be affected. Glossopharyngeal neuralgia resembles trigeminal neuralgia, but it is much less common. It occurs as paroxysmal intense pain originating in the throat from the tonsillar fossa. It may be associated with bradycardia and in such cases it is called vegoglossopharyngeal neuralgia. A trial of phenytoin or carbamazepine is usually effective in relieving pain. Brain stem lesions like motor neuron disease, vascular lesions such as lateral medullary infarction or bulbar poliomyelitis can affect these nerves together resulting in bulbar palsy. Posterior fossa tumors and basal meningitis may involve these nerves outside the brain stem. Complete bilateral vagal paralysis is incompatible with life. Involvement of the recurrent laryngeal nerves, especially the left, occurs in thoracic lesions and this produces only hoarseness of voice without dysphagia.

Anxious? Irritable? Trouble Sleeping? Turn your Vagus On!

What do anxiety, irritability, indigestion, and sleeplessness have in common?

If you said stress, you're on the right track. More specifically, they all result from a lack of Vagus activity. No, not that kind of Vegas. This kind of Vagus is absolutely essential to your health and well-being.

In this chapter, you'll learn why your Vagus nerve is so critical and how to activate it to calm your nerves, rest and digest better, and support your body's natural healing powers.

Your Vagus nerve connects your brain with your heart, gut, and all your internal organs. In fact, its influence is so pervasive that it has been called "the captain" of your parasympathetic nervous system-which is your body's natural relax, rebuild, and repair response team.

Proper functioning of your Vagus nerve keeps chronic inflammation in check, putting the brakes on all major diseases. It regulates your heartbeat, maximizing heart rate variability which is a major marker for heart health. And, it signals your lungs to breathe deeply, taking in the oxygen that replenishes your vital energy.

Your Vagus nerve also translates vital information from your gut to your brain, giving you gut instincts about what is beneficial or harmful for you. Then, it helps you consolidate memories, so you remember important information as well as your good intentions.

Finally, your Vagus nerve releases acetylcholine which counters the adrenaline and cortisol of your stress response, and activates your body's natural Relaxation Response, so that you can relax, rest, and let go.

So, now you have a picture of why activating your Vagus nerve is so critical.

The problem is that our current culture encourages us to be so hyperbusy, so hyperstimulated, that we run in stress mode pretty much all the time, without even knowing it. We are so used to stimulation, that we don't know what true relaxation feels like, much less how to do it.

Instead of practicing a natural rhythm between activity and rest, we are hyperactive. And, we are so conditioned this way that we feel guilty if we're not always doing something or bored if we're not being stimulated and entertained!

As a result, anxiety, irritability, and sleeplessness are constant companions. This prevents us from resting deeply and sets us on the path for chronic illnesses, such as cancer.

So, how can we break this dangerous pattern?

26

Fortunately, your body is highly resilient. It is just waiting for you to activate your natural balance and that is as close as a few slow, deep breaths away.

When you breathe slowly and deeply, your Vagus nerve is activated. It sends calming signals that slow your brainwaves and heart rate, and set in motion all the rest and repair mechanisms of your body's natural Relaxation Response.

So, slow deep breathing is vitally important. But, there's an issue. Living in constant stress mode promotes a pattern of restricted, rapid, shallow breathing.

So, slow deep breathing may take a little practice. Here's a great way to do that:

A Simple Deep Breathing Meditation:

Lie on your back and lightly close your eyes. Rest your hands, one on top of the other, on your lower abdomen.

As you inhale, allow your lower abdomen to gently rise, as if it is filling up with your breath. As you exhale, allow your lower abdomen to relax downwards, as if it is emptying out.

Settle into a nice easy rhythm, lightly following your breath, as your abdomen gently rises and falls. See if it's possible not to force this to happen, but to just pay attention as it happens naturally, easily, effortlessly.

As you continue, see if you can notice the moment you begin to inhale and follow it all the way until you naturally pause. Then, notice the moment you begin to exhale and follow it all the way until it you naturally pause.

Enjoy this soothing rhythm for at least a few minutes and then notice how good you feel.

If you can, go ahead and give this a try right now, so you experience it for yourself...

You can practice this simple deep breathing meditation once a day to release the stress of the day and the layers of tension accumulated from the past. You can do it lying in bed at night before sleep, to prepare your body to rest deeply.

In no time at all, you'll have reset your body's natural balance, and this will translate into living a more balanced, happy, and peaceful life.

Cranial Nerves Mnemonic

You can use a cranial nerve mnemonic to remember the pairs of nerves, but you can also use it to remember other things. Mnemonics are words that you put together that stand for something else. In cranial nerves is could be "Ottafvgvsh" (even though that is not really a word) oculomotor nerve, the optic nerve, the olfactory nerve, the trochlear nerve, the trigeminal nerve, the abducens nerve, the facial nerve, the vestibulocochlear nerve, the glossopharyngeal nerve, the vagus nerve, the spinal accessory nerve, and the hypoglossal nerve. Some might remember it better using three "o's". It's all in how you memorize it. If it makes sense to you that is all that matters.

Cranial nerves mnemonic is how you are going to want to train your brain to remember. If you use this method often you will find that you can often associate other things with the information that you need to remember. The more you do it, the better you will become, but it is good strategy for recalling large amounts of information; especially for tests or exams.

This is not the only way to recall information, but it does work. There are other methods that you can use to retrain your brain to work more efficiently. Some of them are by using lists and mnemonics to help you remember, and others will show you a completely different way of storing information. I'm sure we have seen the kids learning math a different way and actually doing much better with it. Your brain in the same; you can retrain it and make it more effective.

Facts

Depression knows no barriers. It can strike anyone, anywhere and anytime. While the standard treatment for depression is medications, including depressants, selective serotonin reuptake inhibitors (SSRIs) and serotonin norepinephrine reuptake inhibitors (SNRIs), as well as therapies, such as cognitive behavioral therapy (CBT), talk therapy and group therapy, sometimes, a patient doesn't respond to the treatment.

Under severe mental strain, the depressed individual then takes recourse to electroconvulsive therapy (ECT) where electric signals are sent through the brain. These help to sort out chemical imbalances that caused the mental health condition. But under extreme circumstances, even ECT provides no relief or only temporary respite and may result in a relapse. Vagal nerve stimulation (VNS) therapy, primarily used in controlling epileptic seizures, is fast proving to be a sought after treatment for those who do not respond to the traditional mechanisms.

Understanding VNS therapy

The premise of VNS is simple. It works on the vagus nerve, which is the longest cranial nerve in the human body passing from the neck to the thorax and the abdomen. This nerve plays a crucial role in monitoring key functions in the human body. In case there are variations such as increased breathing, the vagus nerve relays messages to the brain regarding how to respond. During VNS therapy, the care giver inserts a small gadget similar to a pacemaker below the neck which activates the nerve.

Skepticism regarding the benefits of the therapy has remained among the medical fraternity, though its function as a placebo has been disapproved by psychiatrist Prof. Hamish McAllister-Williams from Newcastle University. Though he admits that not much is known about its efficacy in cases of severe depression that remain unresponsive to traditional treatments, he is sure that the impact of VNS is not akin to a placebo. Placebo is immediately activated and ends quickly, whereas VNS takes six months before its impact can be felt.

In a 2013 study on depressed patients who were resistant to treatment, it was observed that those who were provided adjunct VNS along with routine treatment for depression, the response rates were higher than when one only depended on treatment as usual (TAU). Another study by psychiatrist Scott Aaronson also revealed that VNS when used with TAU had better long term outcomes than in case of only TAU.

Commenting on the study outcome, Aaronson said, "The tolerability of the device is terrific. The main side effect is hoarseness because the recurrent laryngeal nerve [that supplies the voice box] comes off the vagus nerve." He suggested that the side effects could be controlled by temporarily turning off the device by holding a magnet over it.

Apart from hoarseness in the voice, the therapy also causes frequent coughs, breathing difficulties and changes in heart rhythm. It may also result in one's depression or mania getting aggravated. Therefore, it is necessary to exercise caution before recommending bioelectric therapies for depression.

Alternative treatments for depression

There are many novel therapies for combatting depression. Their use with standard treatments is extremely effective for keeping the condition under check. Three such therapies that engage one's thoughts constructively while keeping negative thoughts at bay are as below:

Art therapy: One can engage in creative arts even without having a prior experience in dance or drama. These activities open the body and mind to a different experience and help one connect to him/her self. They help release all negativity and boost confidence thereby reducing symptoms of persistent sadness and low mood, characteristics of depression.

Mindfulness therapy: Both mindfulness based stress reduction (MBSR) and mindfulness based cognitive therapy (MBCT) promote emotional well being and awaken positivity. Such therapies focus on being in the present without worrying about the past or future. They encourage a person to get attuned to one's senses and gain better understanding and control of their thoughts and behaviors.

Eco therapy: As the name implies, eco therapy helps one connect with nature. Whether it is through walks in the nature or horticulture, it relies on the potential of the nature to heal, soothe and calm.

Do not let depression mar your life

The World Health organization (WHO) reports that depression is the number one cause of disability worldwide affecting more women than men. However, with proper medication and treatment, one can lead a quality life. It is important to seek advice from a certified mental health practitioner who can diagnose the condition in time and suggest appropriate treatment.

The Accessory Nerve (Cranial Nerve XI) and The Hypoglossal Nerve (Cranial Nerve XII)

The Accessory Nerve (Cranial Nerve XI) is a purely motor nerve and it has two roots-cranial and spinal. The Hypoglossal nerve is also a pure motor nerve and supplies the intrinsic muscles of the tongue.

The Accessory Nerve

This is a purely motor nerve. It has two roots cranial and spinal. The spinal root arises from the anterior horn cells of the upper five cervical segments, and it enters the skull through the foramen magnum. These fibers are joined by the cranial root which arises from the caudal part of the nucleus ambiguous and together they leave the skull through the jugular foramen with the vagus. In the jugular foramen, the cranial root fibers join the vagus to be distributed along with fibers of the vagus to the pharynx and larynx. This part of the nerve cannot be tested separately. The spinal part supplies the sternocleidomastoid and upper part of the trapezius.

Testing: This is limited to evaluation of the motor power of the sternocleidomastoid and the trapezius. The sternocleidomastoid is evaluated by inspection and palpation as the patient rotates his head against resistance. The paralyzed muscle is flat and it does not prominently stand out on turning the head to the opposite side. The trapezius is tested by asking the patient to either brace or shrug the shoulders.

The Hypoglossal Nerve (Cranial Nerve XII)

This is also a pure motor nerve and supplies the intrinsic muscles of the tongue. It arises by a series of rootlets from the medulla between the pyramid and the inferior olive, and emerges out of the skull through the hypoglosal foramen before supplying the tongue.

Testing: You should ask the patient to open the mouth without protruding the tongue. In unilaterla paraysis, the tongue curves sliughtly to the healthy side. On protruding the tongue, it is deviated to the paralyzed side. Examine for any wasting or fibrillations of the tongue. This should always be examined without protrusion of the tongue and it indicates a lower motor neuron lesion of the twelfth nerve. In upper motor neuron lesions, the tongue is short and speastic.

Bulbar palsy: This is a syndrome characterized by weakness or paralysis of those muscles supplied by the motor nuclei of the lower brianstem, i.e, the motor nuclei of the ninth to twelfth nerves. In acute lesions as in siphetheria or poliomyelitis, there is no time for muscle atrophy. The chronic forms, as in progressice bulbar palsy or brain stem tumors, result in marked wasting and atrophy of the palate, tongue and sternocleidomastoids. This has to be differentiated from pseudobulbar palsy which is caused by upper motor neuron paralysis of the bulbar muscles as in motor neuron disease and vascular lesions of the upper brain stem.

What Happens in Vagus Doesn't Stay in Vagus

Have you ever wondered if stress at work really can cause you to become sick? The American Psychological Association (APA) says, "Absolutely!" and this is based on the latest research in the field of Psychoneuroimmunology. As you can tell from the long name, this is made up of the study of the psychology (the thoughts of a person), the neurology (the physical paths traveled in the brain), and the immune system all combined in one interactive feedback loop. One of the primary parts of this loop is the Vegus Nerve. Without getting into the medical terminology, basically there are signals sent to the brain when there is an infection or intrusion into the body that is foreign and shouldn't be there. The Vegus sends a signal to the brain that is very similar to the "Threat Response", fight-or-flight, and the brain then sends signals back through the Vegus telling the body how to respond.

Interestingly, what has been discovered is that stress taps into this very same circuit as infection, but starting in the brain rather than the immune system. The APA says that Dr. Steven Maier and his colleagues, who have been deeply studying psychoneuroimmunology, have found that if they stress animals by socially isolating them or giving them electrical shock they see massive increases in the activity in the Vegus.

"Stress and infection activate overlapping neural circuits that critically involve interleukin-1 as a mediator," said Maier.

And, not only does stress produce the expected stress response, it also produces exactly the same behavioral changes--including decreased food and water intake and decreased exploration and physiological changes, including fever, increased white blood cell count and activated macrophages seen in the "sickness response."

"These animals are physically sick after stress," said Maier. "You see everything you see with infection."

What does all this mean to you? "Stress is another form of infection,"said Maier. "And the consequences of stress are... activation of circuits that actually evolved to defend against infection." So, the next time you find yourself feeling "sick", chances are that there has been stress as a precursor to it. The boss that stresses you every time you see them, hear their voice, or even receive an email from them. The pressure to perform and you don't have the confidence that you can get the job done. When you're asked to take on a new assignment or job that either you don't feel qualified for or aren't trained to do. Of course, if losing your job seems likely, the stress level rises significantly!

Consider that stress may play a role with others, too. If your spouse or significant other are sick, you should consider what stress they may have been under prior to becoming sick. Of course, if your children are sick on a continual basis, it could be a clue that there is ongoing stress somewhere in their life. I'm not saying that all sickness is stress related, but there is a reason that we have what are called "disease". Think about it...

The Polyvagal Hierarchy - Rules of Engagement

Ever wonder how the ubiquity of texting will affect our evolution?

Neurophysiologist Stephen Porges, professor of psychiatry at the University of North Carolina, stresses that physiological connectedness is a biological imperative. He proves this by referencing his polyvagal theory which describes the function of the 10th cranial nerve, the vagus.

The vagus is a component of the autonomic nervous system (ANS) which is the system that keeps vital organs like the heart and lungs working. The ANS divides into the sympathetic and parasympathetic systems which spend and renew physiological resources.

Porges suggests we pay attention to the area around the eyes when talking to someone because "physiology determines psychology." If we feel safe when seeing kindness in someone's face, our vagus nerve acts as a "brake" on the heart rate which, without the high vagal tone, would speed out of control. The vagus "inhibits" other behaviors, like talking, which encourages listening.

The vagus nerve arises from two separate nuclei in the brain stem which accommodates older and newer branches. The unmyelinated older branch descends down the back spine and innervates organs below the diaphragm. This "vegetative" vagus is common to all vertebrates including reptiles who freeze when threatened.

The newer myelinated vagal branch descends down the front spine and activates organs above the diaphragm. This "smart" vagus is shared by all mammals. Since mammals are dependent on other mammals to survive, this vagus encourages social engagement.

The 7th cranial nerve controls the face muscles and arises from the same nucleus on the brain stem as the smart vagus. The facial nerve activates the muscles around the eye, including the orbicularis oculi, which registers emotion. Cues we read on another's face track back into the vagus and affect our physiology.

The fight or flight response is part of the newer vagus and arises if we don't see a kind face but a flat face; or we don't hear a prosodic voice but a low monotone. The vagus takes the brake off the heart to mobilize either the fight or flight response. If that system fails and our life is threatened, the vegetative vagus asserts itself and we lose consciousness.

Since the smart vagus controls heart and breathing, respiratory sinus arrhythmia (RSA) measures vagal tone. RSA occurs as heart rate speeds up while inhaling and slows down when exhaling. This variability characterizes a healthy heart.

Greater RSA enhances the calm physiology of the smart vagus and encourages affiliative behaviors like face-to-face contact, listening, prosody and conforming posture. These features help us detect whether we are safe and, if so, supports optimal learning behaviors.

The polyvagal theory is hierarchical: the newer myelinated vagus inhibits sympathetic defenses which inhibit unmyelinated immobilization defenses.

Texting interrupts the "neural exercises" of face-to-face communication so necessary to ground our mammalian nervous system. Lack of practice hinders these rules of engagement. Lose the phone. Reach out and touch someone.

The Yogi's Were Right

In and out, In and out...

It seems simple enough and everyone does it, more than 25,000 times a day in fact.

I'm talking about breathing of course. The most important thing we do every day of our lives. The problem is most people are doing wrong and it is making them sick.

In this post I will shed some light on the importance of breathing and why it's about more than just getting oxygen into our bodies.

But first here's an exercise I want you to try. Don't worry you don't even have to get up.

Exercise:

The 1:2

- I want you to sit up straight. Picture you have a string attached to crown of your head and and it is being pulled toward the ceiling. Poke your chest up and let your shoulders down, Don't force it. Just until it feels comfortable.

- Now relax your jaw and tongue. If you're having a hard time with that, try and swallow- your tongue will naturally relax.

- Now inhale counting to 3 through your nose using your diaphragm. (Your belly should expand before your chest does). To make sure this happens place one hand on your stomach and the other on your chest. When you inhale make sure your stomach moves before you chest.

- Pause at the top of the inhale

- Now exhale counting to 6

- Don't force the air out at the bottom, just let it flow out.

Repeat this for 1 to 2 mins.

How do you feel? Do you feel more relaxed, a little less worried? As you read the rest of the post we're going to explore what just happened while you were "exercising"

What is breathing?

According to Merriam-Webster dictionary, breathing is "to inhale and exhale freely". Now that is true, but it's like saying the Earth is just a rock that revolves around the Sun. Both are true statements, and both are very much lacking in depth.

Let's look a little deeper, shall we? The most important muscle in breathing is the diaphragm. It contracts to create a vacuum in our lungs that pulls air in. It is also the muscle that separates the upper organs (lungs and heart) from the lower organs (liver, kidneys, spleen, digestive and reproductive organs, etc.)

There is a great clip on YouTube that shows the lungs and diaphragm in action. If you're interested please check it out. In that clip the dark pink muscle is the diaphragm and the light pink organs are the lungs. You can see how the diaphragm moves down allowing the lungs to expand the chest and create room for the incoming air. We also have other muscles that work to help us breath. Muscles in our neck, chest and back all work together to perform this vital movement. Could you feel all of the muscles working when you did your exercise? Next time you do the exercise try to feel them.

That is breathing. A little bit more than just inhaling and exhaling freely.

Breathing is pumping

We know that when your diaphragm contracts, it moves down toward your pelvic floor. Another interesting thing happens when you inhale properly. All of those other muscles are engaged and you lengthen your spin, making you taller when you inhale. With all of this movement happening the vertebra in your spine and all of your internal organs are actually getting a nice massage and light squeezing. This massage, or pumping, moves out the old

45

blood and lymphatic fluid and allows the new nutrient rich fluids to move in.

So why is this important? If the fluids don't move they become stagnant. I'm sure we've all walked by a gross looking pond or marsh that smelled of rotting organic matter. That pond or marsh is stagnant and in nature when something is stagnant the decomposers move in. Parasites, harsh bacteria and fungus will overwhelm the system if given places to live. We are a part of nature and when we are stagnant those decomposers proliferate in us. One of the most common forms of stagnation in modern humans is constipation and all the complications that causes for people. I'll have to write something up soon about constipation.

In short breathing is pumping.

The yogi's were right

There are a couple of other cool things that happen in our body, specifically when we breathe through our nose. I will cover them quickly only because I can write an entire post about each one.

You can go back thousands of years and study practices like yoga, tai chi, qi gong, many forms of martial arts and one of the few consistencies all these practices have in common is very precise breathing structures. Inhaling through the nose is the most potent consistency. All of the Masters understood that there was a benefit to breathing in through your nose. Being so in tune with their body provided them this feeling. And in 1998 three Americans won the Nobel Peace Prize proving the Masters right. They won the prize for their studies of nitrogen monoxide or NO. One of the things they discovered about NO was that it is a vasodilator. Which simply means: NO makes the walls of your blood vessel relax, allowing for more blood flow. Alone this study is amazing, but doesn't directly connect to breathing. But then in 2002 a Swedish research group found that NO is formed and released in the human sinuses. They also discovered that if you make a buzzing or ohm sound the concentration of NO increases as much as 15 times. This happens because of the vibration created, from the sound, which mixes the sinus air with the incoming nasal air. These findings led to an experiment that discovered that blood is oxygenated 10-15% more, when you breathe through the nose compared to breathing through your mouth.

To summarize for the folks that don't enjoy this type of information like I do. When you breathe through your nose the NO or Nitrogen monoxide, we produce in our sinuses, goes with the inhaled air into the lungs where it makes the blood vessels around the alveoli expand more. This allows more blood volume to pass over the alveoli which in-turn leads to more oxygen being absorbed into the blood. Don't you just love when science finally catches up with what we know intuitively!

The Vagus Nerve

The nervous system... The most complex system humans know of in the universe. There are trillions of cells in the body constantly communicating back forth with one and other about everything. They communicate about the amount of water they have, the temperature, if they are sick, the list goes on and on, and we are still discovering so many more ways our cells communicate. It really is amazing to think about. It's so fascinating but I digress.

OK so, you have two branches of your autonomic nervous system. They are in charge of things like your respiration, heart rate, digestion, etc. Stuff you don't really think about. One branch is the parasympathetic nervous system or "Rest and Digest" I'll just call it your rest system, and the other is the sympathetic nervous system or "fight or flight" I'll call this your survival system. Both are important and needed but I've noticed that most people spend far too much time in the survival state. It's great when you trip and are about to fall, or when that cat runs across the road while you're driving, but not so good when you are trying to get all of the nutrition out of the food you just ate, or trying to rest. The good news is there are a couple of simple yet effective breathing exercises you can do to stimulate and turn on your rest system, you preformed one of them earlier.

The vagus nerve. Vagus meaning wandering, which describes these nerves perfectly. You have one on each side of your neck. These nerves run from the base of your brain all the way down and connects your internal organs everything from your stomach to your reproductive organs. The unique part about these nerves is that when you breathe properly through your nose (another organ the nerve connects) you activate them and trigger a parasympathetic or rest response in your body. You can put yourself in a relaxed state and gain all the benefits from it. Stimulation of this nerve has been used to treat all sorts of psychological ailments. There have been hundreds of studies done on this nerve and there is tons of information, if you want to do a Google search when you're done reading.

To summarize, belly breathing through your nose stimulates your vagus nerves, which trigger the "rest and digest" portion of your autonomic nervous system.

Phew! You made it through the sciencey part. I love that stuff, but I can understand why some might find it boring and overwhelming. If you enjoyed it I'm glad.

I have another exercise, this one is a little bit more advanced, but I want you to give it a try anyway.

Exercise 2:

The 1:4:2

Get into the same position as the first exercise.

- Again sit up straight. Poke your chest up and let your shoulders down, remember don't force it. Just what feels comfortable.

- Now relax your jaw and tongue.

- Now inhale counting to 3 through your nose using your diaphragm. (Your belly should expand before your chest does)

- Now hold your breath for 12

- Now exhale counting to 6

- Don't force the air out at the bottom, just let it flow out.

Repeat for 1 to 2 mins

But wait!? After I spent all this time telling you to breathe, now I'm saying to hold your breath? Yes! And here is why.

Holding your breath the right way

I stumbled upon the benefits of breath holding while learning to free-dive, because I love spearfishing. Stig Severrinsen is an amazing free-diver and human being. He is THE authority on breath holding on this planet I would write his accomplishments out, but honestly seeing is believing in this case. If you doubt me, look him up when you're done here. And because I find no point in reinventing the wheel I'm going to quote Stig Severinsen's Breatheology website here: "At a first glance holding your breath seems very simple: You inhale, hold your breath as long as you can and then start breathing again. It is also quite a simple measure. How many minutes/seconds? But it is at the same time a multifaceted and complex parameter. It reveals the degree to which you are psychologically in balance - your mental stability - and how finely you are tuned in on your body. The simplicity of breath holds makes it an excellent barometer of your stress level, and makes progress easy to measure... On the long run meditation and breath holds seem to develop your nervous system and brain. Scientific studies have revealed that people who practice meditation and/or freediving show marked changes in their brain and nervous system. One area in the nervous system that undergo changes lies in the brain stem and is connected to the vagus nerve. This is part of the calming parasympathetic pathway which counteracts stress." I don't think I can make it any clearer than that. There is a reason some of the top athletes and CEOs in the world are starting to explore breathe control.

A little saying I tell my clients. To control your breath is to control yourself.

All of this information is to show you how breathing properly really can start you on the path to a healthier life. The exercises I've shown you here are very simple. Please don't let the simplicity fool you though. They are very effective. Plus you don't need any special equipment to do these exercises, and you can do them anytime, anywhere. As you progress in your training you can find many other exercises. If you are ready to dive head first than do some research on Pranayama, the practice of controlling the breath.

Can Chiropractic Help with Asthma?

Bear with me on this one; I've not gone all new age and pseudo-science. But this is worth a second look.

Approximately 300million people worldwide have been diagnosed with asthma, mostly in developed countries. Surprisingly, asthma is considered responsible for up to 250,000 deaths annually. That's a very serious tally for something that is widely misunderstood as a bit of wheezing.

Asthma is defined as chronic (long-lasting) inflammation of the airways. The severity of this varies over time and with external factors, causing fluctuating degrees of wheezing, breathlessness, fatigue, coughing and so forth.

Currently asthma is treated with steroids administered via an inhaler. In severe or long-standing cases, and where co-morbidities exist, these may be used prophylactically. Possible allergens and irritants are also investigated as removable triggers.

For years small numbers of chiropractors have been claiming to be able to treat asthma using spinal manipulation. They state that spinal subluxations (used to mean mal-position rather than partial dislocation) are a major component of disease, including asthma, preventing the body from repairing itself by impinging on "neurological flow".

Frankly, these chiropractors have been widely ostracised for prattling absolute jibberish and fleecing patients out of loads of money.

Research on the topic tends to indicate this was a good move by the chiropractic profession; In its naturally conflicting way, current research neither advocates nor condemns chiropractic treatment for asthma, citing lack of evidence.

Of the existing studies, most are poorly designed and the majority conclude that chiropractic and sham-chiropractic treatments have the same outcomes for asthma patients.

For years small numbers of chiropractors have been claiming to be able to treat asthma using spinal manipulation. They state that spinal subluxations (used to mean mal-position rather than partial dislocation) are a major component of disease, including asthma, preventing the body from repairing itself by impinging on "neurological flow".

So that's a no then? Chiropractic cannot help asthma.

Well, hold the phone. There's more.

Out of curiosity, while treating asthmatic patients for other complaints I have been asking whether their asthma symptoms have changed. Remarkably, all those asked have reported dramatic improvement, and even complete regression, of symptoms.

Alongside this, and with the help of a couple of willing asthmatics, I am running a small case series (to be published at a later date). So far, all cases have demonstrated quite incredible improvement in reported symptoms.

Clearly, jumping to conclusions at this time would be ludicrous; however, some basic physiology may actually explain these observations.

During an asthma attack, inflammation, increased mucus secretion, and smooth muscle spasm constrict airways in the lungs. These are automatic actions in response to a stimulus. This stimulus can vary, but may be increased dopamine, cortisol and adrenaline levels resulting from heightened stress, or something as simple as dust or smoke.

Just for simplicity, we'll leave stress to one side for a moment.

Stimuli, such as dust, are detected by nerves within the posterior pulmonary plexus (a group of nerves in the lungs). This information is then relayed to the thoracic sympathetic chain (another collection of nerves), which then communicates with the spinal cord.

The levels of the spinal cord receiving this input are in the upper thoracic spine (T1-5). The spinal cord then relays this information to the brain, which stimulates increased mucus production, bronchial spasm etc, via the vagus nerve.

Crucially, in normal cases, the nerves in the pulmonary plexus only activate when stimulation is great enough to represent a threat. This is controlled by a neurological mechanism called "threshold", whereby a certain degree of stimulation is required before a message (called an action potential) can sent.

Inadequate stimulation means no message is sent, and this is termed a failed initiation. A series of failed initiations have the effect of sensitising a nerve, meaning that less future stimulation is needed to generate an action potential. This is known as sensitisation and means normal stimuli can activate a nerve. In the case of asthma patients, an example could be cold air triggering bronchial constriction.

The process of sensitisation is very common, contributing to a wide range of painful conditions. In conditions such as carpal tunnel syndrome, for example, up to 85% of cases are attributed to nerve sensitisation.

Typically, postural or degenerative changes within the spine exert physical pressure on adjacent nerves causing continual failed initiations. As a result, normal stimuli become sufficient to generate an action potential, most often perceived as pain.

Within the lung, however, these stimuli are interpreted as irritation, leading to the protective responses we describe as an asthma attack.

Treating postural changes (using primarily upper thoracic spinal manipulation) removes a source of nerve stimulation, thus requiring more stimulation for it to signal again. Decreasing the responsiveness of nerves within the lung means that normal stimuli such as cold air are not perceived as threatening and are less likely to cause an asthma attack.

Chiropractic treatment helps a number of conditions by the same principle, with sciatica and thoracic outlet syndrome obvious examples. Having looked at the comparable anatomy and physiology, it doesn't seem a vast leap to expect results when treating asthma.

There are, however, some flaws with this theory:

Most significantly, it does not take into account the afferent (sensory) role of the vagus nerve. The vagus nerve is involved in autonomic responses, giving the urge to cough when stimulated. While the importance of afferent vagus nerve activity has not been determined in relation to asthma, it is not affected by chiropractic treatment and so may remain a cause of symptoms.

It is also over simplistic to assume that all asthma cases are due to sensitisation of pulmonary nerves. Asthma is a multi-factorial disorder and the treatment of postural changes may not have any impact at all on symptoms.

As mentioned earlier, I have been "experimenting" with asthmatic patients in a very informal way with some very positive results. While the results are virtually meaningless due to lack of scientific rigour, it does seem there might be a plausible (if not water-tight) reason for these observations.

But if the neurological argument does not stack up, what else could be responsible for patient reported improvements?

The word that is most likely to be on most people's tongues (and mine!) is placaebo. This is a striking phenomenon in which patient belief affects outcome, and has been attributed with some startling effects. In all likelihood this plays a major part in any improvements in asthma symptoms, perhaps being the sole cause.

Stress is also an interesting factor to discuss here. It can precipitate asthma attacks, as well as exacerbate them and increase a person's sensitivity to irritants. Stress comes in many forms, but taking time out of your day to see a chiropractor can be a very stress relieving thing. There is also something uniquely reassuring in being able to talk at length about how your complaint affects you, undergoing a full, hands on examination, and subsequently having your condition and potential treatment explained in depth.

A final potential factor in asthma response to chiropractic treatment is the mechanical effect manipulation has on the thoracic cage. Costovertebral (rib) and intervertebral (spinal) joints should articulate with every breath. Due to a variety of reasons, it is exceptionally common for some of these joints to articulate poorly. This makes breathing harder, leading to recruitment of accessory respiratory muscles which enhance the problem, with an overall effect of decreased lung capacity and efficiency. Freeing up these stiff joints with manipulation allows air to be inhaled/exhaled more easily.

In all likelihood all of the factors discussed above contribute in cases where asthma symptoms improve with chiropractic treatment. This, combined with the multifactorial nature of asthma, means that seeing a chiropractor may not help every time or ever completely you're your asthma.

The Second Brain and Mastery of The Human Vehicle

The body's second brain is often referred to as the Enteric Nervous System (ENS). There are hundreds of millions of neurons connecting the cranial brain to the second brain. This is the part of the nervous system that controls and monitors the entire gastrointestinal system from the esophagus to the anus. The really important thing to remember is this. The second brain or enteric nervous system is so extensive that it can act autonomously, with the discovery that if the main connection with the brain - the vagus nerve - is severed the ENS remains capable of coordinating digestion without input from the central nervous system. The second brain and cranial brain are of course in constant communication, however, as the Taoists understand and scientist are beginning to comprehend the second brain is about pure or primal awareness. It is absolutely essential that we bring daily focus into this centre if we are to bring balance back into our bodies and mastery of our human vehicles. Unfortunately as we age we become more disconnected from the gut and second brain preferring instead to constantly be "in the head". On a superficial level this can be seen when we exercise the mid section less and accumulate fat in this area as a "protection" against life or perhaps more appropriately as a protection against our perceptions of life. It is further demonstrated by our lack of

60

correct breathing techniques often chest breathing instead of abdominal breathing which has a catastrophic effect on the body in the long term.

Our cranial brain performs complex computations and rational thinking. Our second brain gets messages from both our external and internal environment which it sends back to our cranial brain. Unfortunately these messages are often ignored much to the detriment of our bodies and the smooth running of our lives. We often fall back into the rational of the mind. Ignoring these messages of "discomfort" both from our external and internal environment chronically will lead to gastrointestinal issues and mental/emotional issues leading finally to physical diseases.

We now know that the second brain is not just capable of autonomy but also influences the cranial brain. In fact, about 90 per cent of the signals passing along the vagus nerve come not from above, but from the ENS (American Journal of Physiology - Gastrointestinal and Liver Physiology, vol 283, p G1217). However the subconscious "gut instinct" much spoken about is a double edged sword. When we are in complete balance and not in "our heads" the second brain does send signals to the brain that may or may not be acted upon by the cranial brain. Very often and much to our detriment these signals are not acted upon because they contradict the logical and limited mind. When we do move on them we are often pleasantly surprised by the outcome feeling more "connected" to something much greater. Often though the signals coming from "gut instinct" are actually instigated by the cranial brain because of past subconscious programming or cellular memory, and we shut down an otherwise sound intuitive and inspirational idea because of anxiety and fear.

The network of neurons in the gut is as plentiful and complex as the network of neurons in our spinal cord, which may seem overly complex just to keep track of digestion. Why is our gut the only organ in our body that needs its own "brain"? Is it just to manage the process of digestion? Or could it be that one job of our second brain is to listen in on the trillions of microbes residing in the gut? Could it be that this hugely complex ecological system requires a brain to manage it and keep it in balance with both our internal and external environment? The answer is of course yes!!!!

Operations of the Enteric Nervous System are overseen by the brain and Central Nervous System. The Central Nervous System is in communication with the gut via the sympathetic and parasympathetic branches of the autonomic nervous system, the involuntary arm of the nervous system that controls heart rate, breathing, and digestion. The autonomic nervous system is tasked with the job of regulating the speed at which food transits through the gut, the secretion of acid in our stomach, and the production of mucus on the intestinal lining. The hypothalamic-pituitary-adrenal axis, or HPA axis, is another mechanism by which the brain can communicate with the gut to help control digestion through the action of hormones.

The second brain also shares many features with the first. It is made up of various types of neuron, with glial support cells. It has its own version of a blood-brain barrier to keep its physiological environment stable. It produces a wide range of hormones and around 40 neurotransmitters of the same classes as those found in the brain. In fact, neurons in the gut are thought to generate as much dopamine as those in the head. Another interesting fact is that about 95% of the serotonin present in the body at any time is in the ENS. Best known as the "feel-good" molecule involved in preventing depression and regulating sleep, appetite and body temperature, seratonin is another important neurotransmitter transmitting signals in the second brain. But its influence stretches far beyond that. Serotonin produced in the gut gets into the blood, where it is involved in repairing damaged cells in the liver and lungs. It is also important for normal development of the heart, as well as regulating bone density by inhibiting bone formation (Cell, vol 135, p 825).

Serotonin is also crucial for the proper development of the ENS where, among its many roles, it acts as a growth factor. Serotonin-producing cells develop early on in the ENS, and if this development is affected, the second brain cannot form properly. This can happen in a child's earliest years due to gut infection or extreme stress and may have the same effect. Later in life this could lead to irritable bowel syndrome, a condition characerised by chronic abdominal pain with frequent diarrhoea or constipation that is often accompanied by depression. The idea that irritable bowel syndrome can be caused by the degeneration of neurons in the ENS is lent weight by recent research revealing that 87 out of 100 people with the condition had antibodies in their circulation that were attacking and killing neurons in the gut (Journal of Neurogastroenterology and Motility, vol 18, p 78).

So can a person's mood be influenced by the nerve signals coming from the gut? Yes of course, it is absolutely crucial that the second brain is kept in holistic balance. It is clear that nerve signals from the gut area is affecting mood. Indeed, research published in 2006 indicates that stimulation of the vagus nerve can be an effective treatment for chronic depression that has failed to respond to other treatments (The British Journal of Psychiatry, vol 189, p 282).

There is further evidence of links between the two brains in our response to stress. The feeling of "butterflies" in the stomach is the result of blood being diverted away from it to your muscles as part of the fight or flight response instigated by the brain. However, stress also leads the gut to increase its production of ghrelin, a hormone that, as well as making you feel more hungry, reduces anxiety and depression. Ghrelin stimulates the release of dopamine in the brain both directly, by triggering neurons involved in pleasure and reward pathways, and indirectly by signals transmitted via the vagus nerve.

Physiological Benefits of Meditation

It is no secret that meditation has its primary origins in eastern philosophies. Indeed, meditation can be traced as far back as 5000 B.C. in Hinduism. But the practice of meditation can be found in many religious traditions, including Christianity and Islam. In Christianity we know it as "prayer", especially the ritualistic forms of prayer such as the rosary and the Adoration in Catholicism. As late as 1975, Benedictine monk, John Main, re-introduced a form of meditation characterized by a repetitious chant of a prayer-phrase. In 1991, the World Community for Christian Meditation was founded.

New Age, an outgrowth of the hippie-counterculture and the astrological coming of the "Age of Aquarius" of the '60s and '70s, synthesized contemporary western ideas of science (psychology) and ecology with Yoga, Hinduism, and Buddhism. Because New Age was/is more of an individualized spiritual movement than an organized religion, it significantly contributed to a wider, more secular acceptance and practice of meditation. The increasing recognition and validation of the benefits of Yoga have resulted in an increasing number of secularized Yoga training centers, not so much as a religious practice but more as a body/mind fitness regimen. Many fitness and exercise clubs offer Yoga and Yogic fitness classes in addition to their physical exercise classes. My wife is a certified instructor in a Body Training Systems (BTS) program called Group Centergy, a synthesis of Thai-chi Yoga and Pilates. The increased popularity of Yoga and its symbiotic relationship with meditation have by mere association contributed to an increased secularization of and familiarity with meditation in the mainstream of contemporary western culture.

With the ever-increasing recognition of life-style induced psychological stress and its negative side effects on health and longevity, the medical disciplines have taken a closer look at the long-professed benefits of meditation. This has been accompanied by an increased interest and acceptance in ancient non-western medicine (sometimes grouped in the category of "alternative medicine"). As early as the 1920's western physicians were making scientific correlations between reduction of muscular tension and reduction of anxiety. In the 1960s, Dr. Ainslie Meares published Relief Without Drugs, a secular treatise on Hindu relaxation techniques to reduce stress and chronic pain. In 1975, Dr. Herbert Benson wrote The Relaxation Response, an expansion of the same subject. Today, Yogic meditation is common in western theories of counseling and psychotherapy. But more interestingly, medical research is finding more and more scientific evidence of the physiological benefits of meditation.

We know that undue physical and psychological stress can have short and long term negative consequences on our health and our longevity. Our contemporary culture is looking for more and more for ways to "decompress". But with our modern lifestyles under accelerated two-income-family financial pressures it's difficult to find the "down time" from the negative stressors. Certainly, weekend escapes from our multi-tasking lifestyles provide short-term relief. And the annual vacation to the slower pace of the tropics (if we can afford it) may lower our blood pressure for a while. But how often do we hear about a friend that arrived home from their vacation more exhausted than when they departed. It seems we are so conditioned to our activity-packed lives that even when we escape, we tend to plan our vacations as if we were in one of those shopping spree contests, frantically running from one tourist attraction to another making sure we get our money's worth.

The question is, how can we reduce and counteract the effects of stress in our everyday lives?

There are everyday proactive strategies for de-stressing. For starters, there is scientific medical evidence supporting the benefits of singing, laughter, and meditation. Not only can these activities reduce stress, they can significantly strengthen our immune system. For the sake of simplicity, let's consider the physiological benefits of meditation.

Our mind in concert with our vagus nerve, the primary monitor of infection throughout our major organs, reacts to stress as if it were detecting the pathogen cells of a bacterial invasion. If you had an infected cut on your finger, the mind/body reaction is to send in the white blood cells to fight the battle against the infection. Our finger at the point of the cut inflames - turning red, swelling, and radiating heat. Under stress, the vagus nerve can over-react telling the brain to defend our primary organs and our cardiovascular system.

When our vagus nerve detects the tension in organs associated with stress, it tells the brain to send in the troops to fight the battle as if we had an invading infection, the same way our immune system will order a response to the infected cut on our finger. This leads not only to increased stomach acid and inflammation but also to the inflammation of the linings of our arteries making us more susceptible to arterial sclerosis and stroke.

It has been found that meditation helps to calm the overly sensitive vagus nerve and shuts down the physiological mechanism that causes these types of inflammation due to stress. Meditation does not eliminate the stress. It alleviates our physiological reaction to the stress. It can also reduce our level of pain.

We certainly know our body's need good quality air rich with oxygen to function at its best. Football fans have seen players sitting on the sidelines breathing supplemental oxygen to restore their depleted oxygen due to the demands of the physical exertions, especially in cities at higher altitudes such as Denver. You may have noticed that the players inhale deeply through their nose. To increase stamina and endurance, long distance runners inhale through their nose and exhale through their mouth. Obviously, we are should be able to inhale much greater quantities of air (and oxygen) through our mouth. So why would a distance runner or an exhausted footfall player benefit from inhaling through their nose? The reason is not due to an increase in oxygen intake but an increase in nitric oxide (NO) that allows blood vessels to relax and dilate thus increasing overall blood flow. We hear little about this very important but ephemeral gas (it lifespan is mere seconds) that plays a major role in our bodily functions. Nitric oxide, normally in small percentages of the air that we breath, is absorbed only through the lining of our nasal passages. Since it has a very short lifespan in our system, we need to replenish it by breathing as often and as deeply as we can through our nose.

Some exercises of meditation encourage deep inhalation through the nose and exhaling through the mouth. This appears to have quite positive effects in restoring and rejuvenating organ function, especially associated with the cardiovascular system. Improved absorption of nitric oxide through meditative deep breathing acts as a neurotransmitter in the brain, similar to serotonin and dopamine, having a calming effect in reducing stress at the same time it promotes wakefulness. Consequently, this type of meditation is best practiced shortly after awakening from sleep. Nitric oxide also promotes healthy skin and reduces hair loss.

Meditation may not be a cure for baldness, but there is considerable evidence that its benefits in the reduction of stress and increased blood flow contribute significantly in improving immunity to infection and reducing cardiovascular inflammation. Heart surgeons are more routinely prescribing mediation as part of the post-surgery regime for their patients.

One Significant Thing Doctors Forget to Tell you About VNS Surgery

Vagus Nerve Stimulation surgery, a last-ditch effort to control seizures, stirs up a controversy amongst those who have the device implanted. Many patients love the relief from uncontrollable seizures. However, many other patients hate the side-effects caused by the surgery and the devise.

Up to 70 percent of people could have their seizures controlled with prescription drugs. For the remaining 30 percent, surgery may be an option. Epilepsy surgery has many different variations; temporal lobe resection, extratemporal cortical resection, and corpus callosal section.

Besides these radical surgeries, Vagus or Vagal Nerve Stimulation surgery (VNS) implants a VNS pulse generator under the skin of the chest in a surgically created pocket. The electrode is tunneled subcutaneously from a neck incision. The VNS uses electrical pulses delivered to the vagus nerve in the neck which travel up into the brain. The vagus nerve has very few pain receptors and therefore provides a good pathway to deliver signals to the brain.

No one knows why the VNS reduces seizures. Proponents believe that persistent VNS causes changes in brain chemistry that may reduce excitatory amino acids and/or increase inhibitory levels. Patients report that VNS reduces the number, length, severity of seizures, and the length of recovery time after seizures. Some report improved quality of life. "It has been almost three years since my VNS, and the only thing I would have changed is that I would have had it about ten years earlier than I did."

However, one important thing doctors forget to tell you before they implant the VNS in a $23,000 surgery: If you have a heart attack, you can not be treated with an automated external defibrillator (AED). Patients with VNS cannot receive emergency treatment with electrical charges used to restore normal heart rhythm to patients in cardiac arrest

Quitting Smoking and Improving your Digestion

Smoking affects the body in many different ways. The most important effect is that it makes the stomach produce more stomach acid, also called gastric acid. Gastric acid is a necessary element for digesting food. If the gastric acid in the stomach is not strong enough digestion becomes incomplete.

The main purpose of the gastric acid is to begin the breakdown of protein and prepare the breakdown of certain vitamins and minerals for later uptake in the small intestine. With too low acidity the person will get stomach pain from unprocessed food moving through the intestines and in the long run he/she will suffer lack of vitamins and minerals.

In order for the stomach to digest the food it will strive to achieve the level of acidity needed with whatever means it has. If the person is a smoker the stomach will crave a cigarette.

But why do some people have enough acidity while others do not? The reason is that some people have had their vagus nerve pinched during birth or before. The vagus nerve runs from the brain down to the large intestine, and messages from the brain to many of the inner organs are passed through this nerve. If the nerve has been pinched or jammed in the neck during birth, the messages from the brain do not travel freely to the recipient organs. Therefore, the stomach does not get the right signals to produce acid and will have to solve the problem with other means, and that could be through the craving of cigarettes.

So if you want to stop smoking you need to liberate the vagus nerve. Any kinesiologist or chiropractor can do this with a simple little procedure that takes only a few minutes. Afterwards you will feel less desire for a cigarette, and now you can quit without any withdrawal symptoms and without nicotine gum or hypnosis.

With optimal stomach acidity you will also gain a number of positive side effects. You will generally get a better digestion and you will absorb the nutrients better. Some sufferers with Irritable Bowel Syndrome (IBS) will feel an improvement and many people will experience their heartburn disappears.

Because of the better digestion your immune defence will improve and you will experience a decrease in certain allergies, like electrosensitivity and sensitivity towards artificial fibers, like polyester.

Stomach Problems Due to Diabetes Explained

As a diabetic you are probably aware that you are at risk of suffering one or more of the awful health problems this disease can cause... heart disease... stroke... kidney disease... nerve damage... neuropathy of the feet and hands... and damaged eyes due to glaucoma, cataracts and retinopathy.

You can also end up with severe stomach problems. Here's why:

The vagus nerve controls the muscles of the stomach and intestines. This nerve, like the other nerves in your body, can be damaged if you fail to control your blood glucose levels. This condition is called gastroparesis.

When the vagus nerve is damaged, the flow of food through your stomach is interrupted, your digestion slows down, and food remains in your body for much longer than it should. Indeed, the length of time your food takes to be digested becomes unpredictable.

Consequences of gastroparesis

This makes it very difficult to monitor your blood glucose and effectively control the effects diabetes is having on your heart, kidneys, nerves, feet and hands, and eyes.

Gastroparesis often has further extremely unpleasant consequences:

Food stays in your stomach for too long so it spoils and you end up with a bacterial infection.

Undigested food can harden and form a lump (called a bezoar) that blocks your stomach and prevents your food moving into the small intestine.

Your stomach acids backup into your oesophagus and damage your throat, a condition known as acid reflux.

You experience nausea and vomiting. In severe cases, vomiting can leave you dehydrated.

You could feel full quickly when eating and experience abdominal bloating.

You could suffer from malnutrition, weight loss and sever fatigue due to vomiting and/or poor appetite.

Though gastroparesis is more common in persons with type 1 diabetes, persons with type 2 can also suffer from it.

Gastroparesis usually only develops after years of high blood glucose levels. In fact, most type 2 diabetics with gastroparesis will have been diabetic for at least 10 years and have been failing to control their blood glucose levels. As a consequence, they are also likely to have some of the other health problems associated with diabetes.

The best thing you can do is to prevent gastroparesis in the first place... by gaining control of your blood glucose levels before the condition starts developing.

How is gastroparesis diagnosed?

Once your symptoms suggest that you may have gastroparesis, there are various tests that can be performed to confirm a diagnosis. These include tests that employ:

Radioactive substances:

Barium x-ray... you drink a liquid containing barium (aka a barium swallow) which coats your oesophagus, stomach and small intestine and shows up on an x-ray which can be interpreted for gastroparesis.

Barium meal... you eat a meal with barium in it. A series of x-rays will show how long it takes to digest your meal, ie how quickly your stomach empties. Too slow and you have gastroparesis.

Radioisotope gastric-emptying scan... you eat food containing a radioactive substance. If a scan shows that more than half your meal is still in your stomach after one-and-a-half hours then you have gastroparesis.

Intrusive methods:

Gastric manometry... a thin tube is inserted into your stomach through your mouth and throat to measure how quickly your food is digested.

Wireless motility capsule... is a tiny device that you swallow with a meal. Motility describes the contraction of the muscles that propel food through your gastrointestinal tract. The capsule measures the pressure, temperature and acidity of different parts in your gut and sends this data in the form of radio signals.

Upper endoscopy... in which an endoscope (thin tube) is passed down your throat so that the lining of your stomach can be seen.

Stomach biopsy... in which a small sample of tissue is taken from the stomach or small intestine which is examined in a medical laboratory for evidence of gastroparesis.

Non-intrusive methods:

Electrogastrography... is a test in which electrodes are attached to your skin to measure the electrical activity in your stomach which can be interpreted for gastroparesis.

Ultrasound... is a test in which sound waves are used to show the inside of your body.

Unfortunately, once any of these tests confirm that you do indeed have gastroparesis there is no cure. However you can manage the condition and its symptoms.

Diet changes to control gastroparesis

One of the best ways to control gastroparesis is through your diet. There are several things you can do:

Frequency: eat smaller meals but eat more often. Instead of three regular meals a day, eat six small meals. This way you will have less food in your stomach and it'll be easier for the food to leave your digestive system.

Texture: choose liquids, such as soups and broths, and other soft foodstuffs that are easy to digest. For example, eat pureed rather than solid fruit and vegetables.

Fats: avoid foods that are high in fat which tends to slow down digestion.

Diet: follow the beating diabetes diet... ie eat natural, unprocessed foods, mainly plants, that are... low in sugar... low in fat... low in salt... high in fibre... digested slowly... but excluding: all dairy products and eggs. You also need to drink plenty of water, to aid the absorption of the fibre you eat which can tend to slow down the passage of food through your stomach.

These simple adjustments to your diet will get your blood glucose levels under control and should also prevent your gastroparesis from getting any worse.

Treatments for gastroparesis

Certain medications can make gastroparesis worse. These include drugs for high blood pressure, anti-depressants, and certain medications for diabetes. You need to discuss this matter with the staff in your diabetes clinic, to see if you can have them changed.

There are several drugs that can be used specifically to treat either the cause or the symptoms of gastroparesis. However most of them have unwanted side effects.

Certain drugs can help move food along your digestive system:

Metoclopramide ... increases muscle contractions in the upper digestive tract which helps food pass through your digestive system quicker. It may also prevent nausea and vomiting. You take this drug before you eat. Its side effects include diarrhoea.

Erythromycin... an antibiotic, also causes your stomach to push food along. Its side effects too include diarrhoea.

Domperidone... is another drug that increases the transit of food through the digestive system. It can also relieve the nausea and vomiting associated with gastroparesis. Its side effects include headache.

Other drugs can also help prevent nausea and vomiting:

Dimenhydrinate... is an antiemetic used in the treatment of the symptoms of motion-sickness, ie nausea and vomiting. It is available as an over-the-counter antihistamine in most jurisdictions. Its side effects include drowsiness and mucus in the lungs.

Ondansetron... is a drug that blocks the chemicals in your brain and stomach that cause nausea and vomiting. Its side effects include headache, fatigue, and constipation.

Prochlorperazine... is another medication that helps control nausea and vomiting. Its side effects include drowsiness, dizziness, blurry vision, skin reactions, and low blood pressure.

In extreme cases of gastroparesis, surgical intervention may be necessary:

Gastric electrical stimulation... uses a surgically implanted pacemaker-like device (a gastric pacer) with electrical connections to the surface of the stomach that sends brief, low-energy impulses to stimulate the contraction of the muscles that propel food through the stomach. This decreases the duration of satiety and may also help reduce nausea and vomiting.

Feeding tube placement... in extreme cases, a tube can be inserted through the abdominal wall directly into the small intestine. In this case the patient is fed special liquid meals through the tube.

Not a pleasant prospect.

Gastroparesis develops slowly over the years. It can be avoided if you get your blood glucose levels under control and the best way to do this is to follow the beating diabetes diet.

Get Some Natural Relief from Diabetic Autonomic Neuropathy Complications

Diabetic autonomic neuropathy (DAN) is a complication of diabetes that affects the entire autonomic nervous system [ANS] causing significant negative impact on both survival and quality of life. Because the ANS serves the major organ systems of the body (e.g., cardiovascular, gastrointestinal, genitourinary, sweat glands, or eyes), any disorder affecting it is experienced as a body-wide dysfunction in one or more organ systems.

The ANS which is responsible for the involuntary functions of the human body is made up of the parasympathetic nervous system which controls the dynamic state [homeokinesis] of the body at rest to regulate the body's "rest and digest" functions while the sympathetic nervous system controls the body's responses to a perceived threat as in the "fight or flight" or emergency response.

The vagus nerve controls the lungs, heart and digestive tract thereby influencing the primary functions of breathing, speech, keeping the larynx [voice box] open during breathing, sweating, monitoring and regulating the heartbeat, satiety, and emptying of the stomach. Thus, when diabetes damages to the vagus nerve it causes loss of innervations and physiologic functions to the anatomic parts of the body it serves.

The esophageal dysfunction in DAN is directly related to vagal neuropathy. The main effects involve swallowing difficulties and heartburn. The heartburn is due to a relaxation of the esophageal sphincter which allows stomach contents to backup into the esophagus causing a burning pain in the chest following eating, bending down and or while lying down at night.

Today's food technology developments have allowed for the development of blenders that we can use to do the 'chewing' of food for us. We can use these blenders to make 'smoothies' which require minimal effort to swallow. This puts less demand on esophageal muscles during swallowing and thereby mitigates the effects of DAN.

Every cell in the human body is primarily designed to run on metabolizing glucose, the end product of carbohydrate digestion to meets its energy requirements. Thus, intimate knowledge of carbohydrate metabolism can help us manage the process from its intake to elimination. Carbohydrates have the advantage of a high fiber content which slows down the rate of glucose absorption to avoid blood glucose overwhelm. Modifying carbohydrate intake by making smoothies out of vegetables and fruits significantly helps us up our raw vegetable intake which helps manage blood sugar.

Autonomic neuropathy in diabetics slows the emptying of stomach contents, due to a partial paralysis [gastroparesis] which in turn leads to other problems such as fermentation of food in the stomach. Diabetic gastroparesis is diagnosed in about 25% of diabetic patients. Typical symptoms are premature feeling of satiety, nausea, vomiting, regurgitation, abdominal fullness, epigastric pain and anorexia. When the food is processed is such ways that allows it to be easily digested and released, the usual presentation of pain associated with it are ameliorated.

The gastric signs of DAN arise from a dilation of the stomach plus the retention of its content. This dilation of the stomach interferes with satiety feedbacks to the brain especially in cases where there is severe acidosis or coma. Green smoothies generally have alkaline pH; this will neutralize the acidosis to prevent the premature satiety feedback to the brain.

Constipation when it is observed is often associated with the compaction and compression of food into hard pellets which can create problems of absorption in the intestine and subsequently form hardened feces. When we employ a blender to make smoothies, the vegetables and fruits are thoroughly chewed allowing for easy digestion and prevent constipation.

DAN causes diffuse and widespread damages of peripheral nerves and small vessels. This is critically important because it is at the level of these small blood vessels called capillaries that transfer of nutrients from the blood to the cells occur. Stabilizing blood sugar will minimize the damage to peripheral nerves and blood vessels.

Individuals with DAN tend to have increased heart rate of 120-130 beats per minute compared to about 60 to 100 times per minute for normal persons at rest. Increased heart rate is associated with dizziness, lightheadedness, angina (chest pain) and shortness of breath. Another symptom experienced by diabetics with DAN is a postural hypotension in which the subject experiences a head rush or dizzy spell upon standing up or stretching. The combined cardiovascular responses mean the diabetic would have a slow reaction time designed to avoid precipitating a critical episode when responding to emergency events around him or her.

Another feature commonly associated with DAN is one of exercise intolerance in which the patient is unable to do physical exercise at the level or for the duration that would be expected of someone in his or her general physical condition. Healthcare providers very often advice diabetics to alter their lifestyle which is a euphemism for exercise. One hears phrases like 'don't be a couch potato' thrown around often but the physiological presentations of postural hypotension and exercise intolerance explains why persons with DAN show no interest whatsoever in taking up the exercise advice.

How to Increase the Acidity and Improve your Digestion

The hydrochloric acid in the stomach is one of the most important factors for proper digestion. The acid has a number of functions and if these are incompletely performed, the person will in the short term experience acid reflux, stomach pain and indigestion. In the long term he or she may suffer IBS, food intolerance, food allergy, vitamin and mineral deficiency and even some autoimmune diseases.

The main functions of the acid are to initiate the breakdown of proteins, vitamins and minerals. The acid also kills bacteria and parasites so they don't reach the intestines and the bloodstream.

With too low acidity the food will stay longer in the stomach before it can continue and while the stomach struggle to digest the food (the stomach is a muscle), it can force some liquid up the esophagus. This is what people feel as heartburn (also called

GERD). If the acidity level had been higher the valve between the stomach and the esophagus would not have opened.

During the extended time the food stays in a stomach with low acidity the person will suffer bloating.

When the semi-digested food continues to the small intestine, further digestion is complicated because the intestine cannot process it in the form it has. That is when abdominal pain sets in.

Furthermore, the food will contain microscopic, undigested elements that find their way through the wall of the intestine and into the bloodstream. These can cause headache and food intolerance and allergy. This phenomenon is known as leaking gut.

If you have these symptoms and they are caused by too low stomach acidity, taking medicine to lower the acidity further will make the problem worse.

To find out whether you have too low or too high acidity take 1 to 2 tablespoonful of apple cider vinegar before meals. You can either take it directly with a spoon or mix it with a little bit of water in a glass. If this eliminates the heartburn your problem is deficiency of acid production.

It is estimated, that around 90% of people with heartburn or similar problems have too low acidity.

The reason the stomach doesn't produce acid enough is because messages from the brain to the stomach are blocked. The brain sends messages to the stomach (and other organs) through the vagus nerve. This nerve starts in the brain and passes down the neck all the way to the intestines. With some people this nerve was pinched in the neck during birth and this blocks part of the messages to the stomach about acid production.

The vagus nerve can be liberated easily by a kinesiologist or chiropractor with a non-invasive little procedure that takes a few minutes. It is worthwhile to take the effort to have this done; your whole digestion will improve. Furthermore, if you are a smoker your craving for cigarettes will disappear and some allergies like electrosensitivity will decrease.

Ten Remedies for Hiccups

Hiccups are those annoying, nerve raking and sometimes even aching reflexes that we have when the vagus nerve or one of its branches, which runs from the brain to the abdomen, is irritated. The causes for hiccups are almost unknown, as none really knows how does the vague nerve get to be irritated. There are nonetheless some suppositions and a few remedies that would treat hiccups when they appeared.

At the bottom of all these rests the assumption that you need to give your brain the impulse that you are doing something important and hiccups need to stop. Thus, most of the remedies try to give your body something else to do.

One of the first remedies we learn about when we get hiccups is to hold our breath or as long as we can or until we sense that the hiccup is gone.

Another one is to eat a spoonful of sugar. It works better if you can put the sugar on the back of the tongue.

Let yourself be surprised. Although pretty dangerous with some older people or if hiccup is determined by a nervous reaction, trying to let someone surprise or scare you might prove pretty useful to stop from hiccups.

Drink some water. Take a little bit of water and drink it. If you can, put some lemon juice in it. Drink it slow, with small sips and make sure it is not very cold.

Sometimes, hiccups may emerge because you are cold, so keep yourself warm. Drink some hot tea and make sure you are well dressed.

Eat slowly. When you eat fast, your stomach has no time to digest and it becomes more easily irritable. Eat slowly and do not eat too much. Try to give your body just the amount of food it needs to stay fit.

Put your fingers in your years. Scientists state that the nerve that makes hiccup appear can extend to the auditory system. So try to cover your ears and put your fingers in your ears; however be gentle when doing this and do not force too much inside.

Another remedy that seems to work is to stick out your tongue and yank on it. It is also kind of fun, so try not too laugh too much, as you might get the reversed reaction and hiccup more.

Tickling is also a good remedy against hiccups. Ask somebody to tickle you in your sensitive spots or use a cotton swab to tickle your soft palate of the roof of your mouth.

Give Birth a Chance

In our culture, birth is unfortunately presented as a scary illness where something can go wrong at any second. If you buy that then you should know that many elderly people die on the toilet due to straining while, well, you know why people strain on the toilet. (This is a result of stimulating the vagus nerve, which causes a big drop in heart rate; not so good if you've got a bad ticker). Why then are people over the age of 65 not strongly advised to go to the hospital or their clinic whenever they have to poo? Because it's ridiculous, that's why. Because it's a normal, natural process...

I firmly believe that healthy pregnant women have the right to have their babies at home or in birth centers attended by midwives. Why is that? This is how they do it in many other areas of the world. But just because everyone else does something doesn't mean we should follow suit, right? Wrong. The United States has higher fetal and maternal death rates than some third world countries and since only 1% of babies are born at home, one can only deduce that this is happening in the hospital. How can this be when we have so much wonderful technology available? It's that technology that gets us in trouble. Women are no longer taught to trust their bodies. We are given the message that we need a machine to tell us when we have contractions or when the baby is ready to come out. Trust me, you know.

Continuous electronic fetal monitoring keeps women strapped to the bed when the only conclusion that has come from numerous studies is that EFM leads to many unnecessary c-sections. Not to mention the fact that all these wires keep women stuck in bed to labor on their backs, which is the MOST uncomfortable position to have your baby in. The only worse position would be to do it upside down. However, if someone were able to profit from it, I'm sure it would be suggested that women give birth that way.

There are other reasons for our terrible statistics: hospital-acquired infections, inducing too early, induction period that causes way too much stress on the baby with harder and faster contractions. Using Cytotec, an ulcer drug used to soften the cervix that has been proven to rupture a woman's uterus and cause fetal death. This of course leads to more epidurals earlier in labor, which leads to exhaustion and higher vacuum and forceps use and c-sections. Not to mention the fact that women aren't allowed to eat when they are about to face the most grueling work their bodies can do. Would you set off on a cross-country road trip on an empty tank of gas? Didn't think so. This used to be done to prevent women from aspirating during surgery but today most women are awake during a c-section and fully aware of when they will be sick.

The domino effect of medical intervention is staggering considering that most of them are completely unnecessary. Birth is a normal, natural process. Women have historically tended to other women during labor and birth. It wasn't until male practitioners came along that everything took a turn for the worse. Don't get me wrong. Doctors are great. Women with high-risk pregnancies need those doctors and the technologies that the hospitals provide. But most women aren't high risk. And the ones that are told they are should really do their research and be fully educated on the reasons for their high-risk classification before they take anyone's word for it. A woman has the right to decide how she wants her birth to go. We need to throw the fear out the window and give birth a chance.

Major Anxiety & Depression

Some people go through brief periods of "the blues" or "anxiety" and others live with either or both for a lifetime.

For those in the second category, there are a number of solutions. No, it won't go away, most likely, but you will get a reprieve for a number of hours and sometimes days.

Obviously traditional therapy with a trained professional should take precedence over all other

modicums of treatment.

However, in my experience, and many others whom have been afflicted with the lifetime experience of GAD (Generalized Anxiety Disorder) and (TRD) Treatment Resistant Depression, there are some activities that can lift both, at least for awhile. And if done often enough, the severity of bouts of either is lessened.

Walk.

That's right. Something as simple as walking. I realize some persons reading this book are wheelchair-bound or have some other disability in which they are unable to walk, but there are plenty of aerobic exercises that "clue" the nervous system that it can "calm down" and a trained professional in that area can be most helpful.

But for those who can walk, but don't want to, still, walk. Don't try to conquer the world with a marathon on the first walk. A few blocks is fine to start if you've not been walking much in the past.

GAD is another story. Yes, the VNS implant helps it somewhat but not totally like it does the depression. Sometimes I have to take medicines for it too. But whether I take them or not, on days I walk, I feel much less anxiety the rest of the day and night, and sleep better. On days I don't walk, even if I take the medicines for anxiety, I feel anxiety to a certain degree. Of course stress and anxiety is a part of life, but that does not mean GAD (anxiety magnified) has to be so.

I take a long walk every day that the weather permits now. To stay in shape, I used to go to the gym, but found I could do crunches and push-ups, etc at home, and it didn't cost me a thing and I stayed in just as good of shape.

There is not a lot of empathy or sympathy for those who suffer from depression and/or anxiety; the two often go together. It is not a disease that is totally socially-acceptable.

Due to school-shootings, insanity pleas after violent crimes, etc. many still stereotype everyone who suffers from either disease to have such violent tendencies (I have never been violent in my life nor wanted to hurt myself). It is more aggravating than painful; though clinical studies have proven that both anxiety and depression can and often does cause physical pain that is inexplainable.

Sometimes the person with the disease is not sure which is more painful, the disease itself, or the social isolation.

My colleagues have often told me to "stay quiet" and "mum's the word" etc. about this ailment, that persons can and will use it against me, and I have much to lose.

I say, "So what? I also have much to gain. If just one person can win the battle against this awful ailment, if someone "uses it against me" it was all worth it.

As I said, in 2001, I suffered a major heart attack. It did not feel very good. But I can promise one thing. If I had a choice of a heart attack a day, or major depression and anxiety, I would choose the heart attack in a heartbeat (no pun intended).

And I am certain others struggling with the same ailment feel the same way. There is no way to explain it.

Fortunately today, modern medicine has a much better handle on it than they did even a decade ago. If you've not explored therapy, exercise and other ways to help yourself, please do. Life is worth it and the chance to be a productive and contributing member of society (I never really was until a decade ago, is well worth the battle). It beats laying in bed until 3pm, that's for sure.

The Parasympathetic Nervous System (PSNS)

Parasympathetic Nervous System The Parasympathetic Nervous System (PSNS) is part of the Autonomic Nervous System (ANS), along with the Sympathetic Nervous System (SNS) and Enteric Nervous System (ENS). Contrary to popular belief, the PSNS and the SNS act together in a complimentary way rather than an antagonistic way. The SNS springs into action when a quick response is required, and the PSNS comes into its own when slower actions are needed.

Typically the PSNS is involved in:

• Salivation

• Lacrimation

• Urination

• Digestion

• Defecation

The ANS, regulates the body's visceral organs via the innervation of 3 kinds of tissues:

• Smooth Muscle

• Cardiac Muscle

• Glands

The PSNS is found in Cranial and Sacral regions of the Spinal Cord and is therefore often described as having a Cranio-Sacral outflow. The SNS for similar reasons is described as Thoraco-Lumbar in outflow. T1 to L2 In the cranium the PSNS originates from the following cranial Nerves:

• Third Cranial Nerve - Oculomotor

• Seventh Cranial Nerve - Facial

• Ninth Cranial Nerve - Glossopharyngeal

• Tenth Cranial Nerve - Vagus

In the Sacral Region the PSNS is derived from spinal nerves

• S2

• S3

• S4

... which are referred to as the Pelvic Splanchnics. PSNS In The Cranial Nerves. Oculomotor Innervates the orbit to control the Ciliary Muscle which is responsible for accommodation and the Sphincter Pupillae Muscle which is responsible for miosis or constriction of the pupil in response to light or accommodation.

Facial Parasympathetic function within the Facial Nerve controls secretion of the Sublingual and Submandibular Salivary Glands, the Lacrimal Gland, and the glands associated with the Nasal Cavity. Glossopharyngeal. Parasympathetic fibers innervate the Parotid Gland. Vagus Vagus gives no Parasympathetic input to the cranium, but several Parasympathetic Nerves leave Vagus as it enters the Thorax. • Recurrent Laryngeal Nerve, which becomes the Inferior Laryngeal Nerve. Each Recurrent Laryngeal Nerve supplies the Trachea and the oesophagus with Parasympathetic Secretomotor Fibres for glands associated with them. • Cardiac Nerves which form the Cardiac and Pulmonary Plexuses around the heart and lungs. As the main Vagus Nerves continue into the Thorax they become intimately linked with the Oesophagus and Sympathetic Nerves from the Sympathetic Trunks to form the Oesophageal Plexus.

The major function of Vagus now is to control of the Gut Smooth Muscles and Glands. The extent of the PSNS in the Abdomen includes the Pancreas, Kidneys, Liver, Gall Bladder, Stomach and Gut Tube.

Pelvic Splanchnic Control The Pelvic Splanchnic Nerves, S-2, S-3 and S-4, innervate the Pelvic Viscera. The tissues in the Pelvis under Parasympathetic control are:

• Bladder

• Ureters

- Urinary Sphincter

- Anal Sphincter

- Uterus

- Prostate

- Vagina

- Penis.

Type 2 Diabetes - Diabetes and Gastroparesis

Gastroparesis is one of the common complications of Type 2 diabetes. It is actually a form of diabetic neuropathy that specifically affects a major nerve which runs from the brain to the colon called the vagus nerve. The vagus nerve is responsible for helping the body move food through the digestive system and process it properly, among other duties. When gastroparesis is present, the vagus nerve is damaged and cannot process food correctly.

Problems can include symptoms of:

nausea,

diarrhea, or

constipation.

Gastroparesis is translated as "stomach paralysis". This perfectly describes what is happening when the vagus nerve is damaged. Gastroparesis is caused by elevated blood sugar levels over long periods of time. As blood sugar remains elevated, it not only damages the blood vessels which supply the vagus nerve but it also damages the nerves by creating a chemical change within them.

When the body begins to experience gastroparesis food is no longer moved through the digestive tract and into the stomach as it should. Once food is in the stomach it isn't digested efficiently and in a timely manner. This means food not only takes much longer to reach the stomach, but once there, it has nowhere to go.

What can this combination of issues cause? When food is allowed to sit without being broken down, two things begin to occur. The bulky material can cause a slew of symptoms from nausea to vomiting. Second, it provides a breeding ground for bacteria to grow which can ultimately result in an infection within the digestive tract.

How is gastroparesis identified? The symptoms include nausea, bloating, abdominal pain and even heartburn, as the food pushes back up into the esophageal tract. This "full" sensation can cause a lack of appetite and as time passes, even weight loss.

The treatment for gastroparesis involves multiple steps. The first, and most important task to take care of is keeping your blood sugar levels under control as much as possible. Once the condition is present this can be rather difficult to accomplish since your food will not be digesting properly. This will naturally result in wild fluctuations in your blood sugar, making it even more difficult to achieve balanced sugar levels.

The next step involves choosing your food wisely. You want to avoid high amounts of fiber and other foods which will require more work for your body to digest. Also, stay away from foods which are not cooked thoroughly and particularly stay away from fats altogether. Eating smaller meals more frequently is another essential step to take.

Type 2 diabetes is not a condition you must just live with. You can take control of the disease, take back your health and prevent developing gastroparesis.

Infantile Colic - Natural Cures that Work for Restless Babies that Can't Sleep

Infantile colic is one of the most common early childhood diseases affecting millions of babies annually worldwide. The condition often demonstrates in the early stages of life following birth. Sign and symptoms of a baby with colic include incessant crying, contracted stomach muscles, difficult nursing, copious amounts of bowel gas, reflux, constipation, and an inability to self-soothe or calm even when held and comforted. Colic can be extremely alarming to parents especially if they are new parents with their first child. So many aspects of early parenthood are unknown and adding a distressed inconsolable baby to their woes is often overwhelming. A lack of sleep for both baby and parents can begin to weigh on the family unit and sometimes parents find themselves emotionally at the brink of collapse and may even suffer with depression and anxiety from their inability to control the situation with their newborn.

One of the prevailing theories explaining the cause of infantile colic is distress to the autonomic nervous system caused by stress to the vagus nerve. The vagus nerve emerges near the base of the skull and courses to the digestive system providing parasympathetic nerve supply for the stomach. At times, during birth or while in-utero, a baby upsets this system through birth trauma or inappropriate position in the uterus or birth canal.

While the baby may have birthed and seemed fine post birth, often the stress to this system has gone undetected. At times, the baby born with cesarian section is often at higher risk because the natural birth actions of baby and mother are bypassed and the strain applied to a baby while birthing through a small insertion in the mother's abdomen can strain the cervical neck area of the child.

A pediatric chiropractor is trained to detect the stress on the vagus nerve through the assessment of a condition called vertebral subluxation. Vertebral subluxation to the top segments of the spine are often the most probable cause of the colic. Through gentle analysis and correction using light movements on the spine and base of the head, most babies will improve within 1-6 visits. The chiropractic physician provides a treatment called adjustments to correct the nerve interference. Other home therapy which provides help for the newborn with colic will include the use of probiotics and digestive enzymes. If a mother is nursing, some subtle changes in her diet will also help in some cases. Removing dairy, gluten, garlic, and spicy foods will often render some aid in the condition of the newborn.

Other home care remedies that can often help include giving the baby frequent epsom salt baths with some baking soda to provide soothing magnesium to the muscular system of the child. This will help calm muscles and nerves in the baby. Frequent attempts to burp the child during feeding can also help in some cases and changing formulas to predigested varieties will also aid in some cases. However, the most effective method for helping a newborn with colic is pediatric chiropractic care.

Various studies have been published substantiating the significant improvements babies will experience with chiropractic care. A parent considering this method of care has very little to worry about and his/her baby has everything to gain. A happy, calm, and content baby is special and experiencing a happy baby can light up a room and make all who know and care for the baby enriched with life and love.

Common Epilepsy Treatments

There are actually many common epilepsy treatments that one suffering from this brain disorder may benefit from participating in. However, the most common form of treatment is drug therapy. This is basically due to the fact that prescription medications have been deemed as the most appropriate course of action for preventing and stopping seizure activity.

The goal of treatment is to reduce the occurrence of seizures and other uncomfortable symptoms associated with epilepsy. When deciding which epilepsy treatments are the most appropriate for your condition, there are many factors that must be considered.

These include the severity of the seizures experienced, if you suffer from other medical conditions, and your general medical history. Here, you will be introduced to several of the common epilepsy treatments.

Medication

Many individuals are put on medication therapy. These medications are in a class of drugs known as anticonvulsants. There are several different drugs that are used to prevent and stop seizures. These include, but are not limited, to the following:

• Neurontin

• Tegretol

- Dilantin

- Lamictal

- Lyrica

- Topamax

The down side to drug treatments for epilepsy is that many uncomfortable and troublesome side effects may be experienced while taking the medications. These side effects may include lethargy, cognitive complications, depression and other types of mood fluctuations, and even thoughts and attempts of suicide.

Nerve Stimulation

A type of nerve stimulation that is identified by specialists called "Vagus" is used as a common treatment for epilepsy. There is a nerve found in the back side of the neck that is relatively large that is called the "Vagus" nerve. Specialists will send short, quick electrical bursts to this nerve so that they reach the brain. While this is not a treatment that has been used for a long time, it is a treatment that is becoming more common as it seems to provide a type of balance within the electrical circuitry of the brain.

The Ketogenic Based Diet

There is a special diet that is low in carbohydrates and exceptionally high in fats that may specialists put epilepsy patients on to treat their condition. This diet works to ensure that the body burns the fat that it receives for energy rather than burning the fat for glucose. This diet has been found to assist individuals in experiencing less seizure activity.

This seems to be effective in patients that suffer from epilepsy due to a metabolic disorder or when the body unsuccessfully processes vitamins and nutrients. Most patients that benefit from this type of epilepsy treatment are children.

It is unknown why this seems to work better for children. The down side to this diet is that it could result in a high level of triglycerides in the body. If you are interested in learning about common epilepsy treatments, be sure to discuss all of your options with a medical professional.

My Kitty's Nervous System

As a trauma therapist, my biggest dread is being responsible for creating trauma for my kitty. I hate trauma which is why I heal it for a living. What I observed today, however, is that when the nervous system is adapting appropriately, it's not so bad.

My kitty was a rescue. She was six months old when I adopted her. When i met her she had a large cone on her head. I noted the rod stuck in her leg keeping her bone set straight and wondered how I would ever nurse her back to health. I was told that she had been hit by a car and the rod was setting the bone until she was ready for surgery. I did nurse her back to health.

Through our ten-year adventure, I have noted that I am not permitted to go any where near her once injured leg. If I move toward it, I watch her tense up and bang her tail furiously as if to say "Stay away from there!" I know that she is not in pain. Curiously, however, she clearly has not forgotten the trauma from her once broken leg. This proves the theory that body remembers and does not forget physical or emotional trauma.

Today was a dreaded adventure. My kitty was sent to the bathroom. Workmen stomped into my house with their noisy tools and banged on the walls. The windows were being replaced. After an hour I went in to visit her. She was unusually friendly and very talkative. Curious and cuddly she was determied to manipulate me to open the door and let her out of this miserable hot bathroom. I wondered if this was her vagus nerve acting up, trying to socially engage her owner due to the horror of what was going on outside the bathroom door. Beyond cuddling, purring, and talking, I knew she was preparing to make a quick get away once that door was opened. She was preparing to flight. I could feel her heart beating furiously. Thinking about ways to regulate the vagus nerve, I began to hum to her. This seemed to help and she resigned to waiting behind the door. Once I opened the door to let her out she slowly moved into the situation, ears pinned, eyes wide open, and tail slightly down. Then a large bang and faster than a speeding bullet she shot off under the bed.

Applying Porges Poly Vagal theory of fight/ flight/freeze, watching my kitty through this lense is quite interesting. Running under the bed to safety was very productive to her nervous system. Minutes later when the chaotic sounds passed she was sitting by the air conditioner quite content. As I watched her, I thought, huh, now that's a healthy adaptive nervous system. Permitted to follow through on the instinct to flight and then being able to control her environment by hiding under the bed where it was safe actually diminished any after effects of locked trauma in her nervous system because she had the freedom to experience flight - ing without being stopped, attacked, or trapped. It was unnecessary to fight and risk becoming hurt and unnecessary to immobilize (freeze). Humans can learn a lot from simply observing their pets nervous system.

More importantly, my kitty's pre frontal cortex is not getting in the way of experiencing any sensation that is necessary for her to orient her nervous system back to the baseline. She isn't going to intellectualize the traumatic experience. She isn't; going to talk herself out of what she felt, or deny her instincts, thus ending up with a throbbing headache, gut problems, or dissociative episodes. She just experiences whatever her instincts tell her to do. The result is a happy content kitty sitting calmly by the air conditioner, roughly five minutes, after the traumatic episode.

Type 2 Diabetes - Digestion and Diabetes

When Type 2 diabetes strikes, almost every system and area of your body is affected at some level... with some systems being disrupted more than others. While some of these areas might only be mildly impacted, it doesn't diminish the fact they are not operating at optimal efficiency. But other areas are much more dramatically impacted. As a result, the person diagnosed with Type 2 diabetes has to not only deal with their diabetes, but the many other life-altering side effects that have been created because of it.

One of these areas which is greatly impacted is digestion. This is due to autonomic neuropathy and involves the nerves whose functions are more or less automatic... those that control:

the stomach,

sweat glands,

digestive tract,

intestinal system,

bladder,

penis, and

circulatory system.

Gastroparesis, a neuropathy-related digestive problem, can include symptoms of nausea, diarrhea, or constipation... to name a few.

Medications can give relief for most symptoms of gastroparesis, as can such simple changes in eating habits as eating smaller meals more often and also adjusting the amount of fiber in your diet.

Also known as paralysis of the stomach, gastroparesis occurs when the vagus nerve, or the central nerve responsible for crushing food into particles which can be easily digested, becomes damaged. Once the vagus nerve is damaged, food is not broken down properly and, therefore, it cannot mix with the appropriate enzymes for processing. This means the stomach doesn't empty normally and naturally, food is then not absorbed. These processes are also impacted negatively by a high-fat meal.

When the normal digestive process is interrupted, the individual will then experience a long list of uncomfortable symptoms. They can have:

diarrhea,

nausea,

abdominal pain,

constipation,

vomiting,

bloating,

a feeling of fullness,

heartburn,

weight loss. or

a combination of some or all of these symptoms.

Even if stomach acids and digestive enzymes are released as intended, they will still contribute to the side effects due to the fact the food has not been adequately processed for digestion.

Unfortunately, this is not the end of the problems as blood sugar levels will also be affected dramatically. When food is unable to be digested, it makes it incredibly difficult to control your blood sugar levels. Since the body is not receiving the necessary vitamins and nutrients from the food, the body is not able to receive what it needs in order to have balanced blood sugar.

But the trouble does not stop there. When blood sugar levels are not balanced, it unfortunately also means the gastroparesis worsens. This ensures the vicious cycle continues. This is why it is important to keep gastroparesis away to start with.

If a person with Type 2 diabetes begins to experience problems as an aftermath of eating, they should consult with their doctor immediately.

Type 2 diabetes is no longer a condition you must just live with. It need not slowly and inevitably get worse. Now is the time to take control of the disease... and take back your health and your life.

Ten Common Symptoms of Parkinson's that Don't Involve Movement

To the average person on the street, and even to most non-neurologist doctors, Parkinson's is a disease mainly characterized by faulty movement and balance. Even James Parkinson, discoverer of the disease, described it in 1817 mainly terms of motor symptoms, the big three classic cardinal findings, still described that way today as tremor, rigidity, and Bradykinesia (slowing) seen in the extremities with one side usually showing worse symptoms than the other during the entire course of the disease.

Ironically, only half of the 10 most common warning signs of Parkinson's disease, designated by the National Parkinson Foundation actually involve motor symptoms. The remaining half involve symptoms that the average person and even actual sufferer might not associate with images of Parkinson's disease. Many of these non-movement symptoms can develop as early as 3-5 years before motor disturbances appear and cause a sufferer to actually end up before a neurologist. Creating a stronger public awareness of some of these non-motor symptoms might bring in more patients for evaluation who would otherwise be dismissed and help patients themselves and even loved ones and family to understand that some of the behavior seen does not arise out of personal laziness, self- pity or any other non-productive behaviors.

Non-motor symptoms derived from the original list of 10 warning symptoms of Parkinson's disease as designated by the National Parkinson's Foundation:

1. a loss in sense of smell

2. trouble sleeping

3. constipation

4. soft or low voice

5. dizziness or fainting

I have added the following two:

1. fatigue and EDS (excessive daytime sleepiness)

2. new-onset depression or anxiety disorder

Interesting Brain details you may skip over.

If you look at areas of the brain affected by Parkinson's disease under a microscope, you see a very characteristic abnormal doodad called a Lewy body. Although the actual nature and cause of these abnormal brain cell units of debris is not known, it seems that somehow the depletion of the brain chemical dopamine to that brain area somehow causes them to develop. Affected cells misfire and eventually die. Without getting into too much detail, my main reason for mentioning this, is that if you look at brains and people with early-stage Parkinson's disease, even in those who have not developed motor symptoms, you find these Lewy bodies. Where they're found directly matches brain regions involved in each of these non-movement-related symptoms.

These Lewy bodies can be found in brain regions affected by Alzheimer's disease also. They consist primarily of an abnormal protein called alpha-synuclein. Investigators are now looking at vaccines that could potentially stimulate the immune system into getting rid of alpha-synuclein from the brain. In the laboratory, when you remove alpha-synuclein, cells that were otherwise destined to die, survive.

In early Parkinson's disease, Lewy bodies can be found in the olfactory region of the brain that processes the sense of smell. They can also be found in an area of the brain stem that controls autonomic function of the G.I. tract (constipation) and which also controls a very important autonomic nerve called the vagus nerve which influences the voice box or larynx (soft or low voice) and the entire cardiovascular system (dizziness and fainting).

You can also find them in a brainstem area that controls alertness and sleep called the reticular formation, and and in an area that supplies the brain with a chemical called serotonin. Depressed and anxious brains have low serotonin.

Back to clinical:

Thus, every single one of the non-motor (non-movement-related) symptoms mentioned can occur and often do emerge early in the disease, and often before any motor changes are seen. Each one can be traced to some abnormal brain region. Other symptoms related mostly to the disruption of the areas that control autonomic function include frequent urination from an overreactive bladder, and sexual dysfunction in the form of erectile dysfunction in difficulty with orgasm.

The degeneration of areas of the brain that control sleep don't merely produce insomnia. The classic sleep disturbance seen in Parkinson's involves falling asleep without much trouble, but waking up one to three hours later and often in a somewhat panicked state.

Type 2 Diabetes - Pain, Referred Pain and Diabetes

Nobody likes pain and it can occur in any part of your body, at any time. However, pain doesn't always originate in the spot where you actually feel it. You often get referred pain. This is when a spot feels painful but the pain is being referred from another point in your body.

For example, if you have neck pain, it may be caused by general muscle tightness in your upper back. If you have a massage, your upper back needs to be worked on as well as your neck, in order to ease the pain. If your neck is the only spot worked on, the pain may ease a little but it will return as the area causing the pain was not attended to.

If you are having a heart attack, you may get referred pain in your neck, arms and shoulder. If you have pain in your throat, that can cause referred pain in your ear. If you eat icy cold food, you may experience what's known as "brain freeze" and this causes a bad headache because the coldness chills your vagus nerve.

If you get referred pain from your spine, it's generally because a nerve or a nerve root has become compressed. Causes include:

muscle spasms,

disc problems,

tumors,

fractures of the spine, or

osteoarthritis.

Referred pain is more common in older people but it can strike at any age. Trauma can cause referred pain for anybody.

Symptoms of referred pain from the thoracic and cervical spine include:

weakness in the muscles, poor coordination, especially in your fingers and hands, tingling and/or numbness in your hands and fingers, and pulsing pain in your chest, arm, shoulders or neck.

Naturally, the actual location of symptoms will depend where the problem originates from. If you put your hands on your head, you may be able to temporarily ease the pain as this increases the amount of space between your cervical vertebrae.

When nerves become compressed, they cannot send out the same messages as they would normally and that's why you may get numbness and tingling. Other nerves carry "motor" function messages and, if affected, your muscles can become weakened and you may find it hard to coordinate your movements properly.

Diabetes makes pain worse because high and unstable blood sugar affects your nerves. This means you can suffer from referred pain more often due to nerve damage.

If you have pain:

consult a physical therapist to help determine the exact nature of the problem and the best means to correct it.

also consider your posture. Leaning over a desk all day, can cause additional pressure on certain parts of your spine, leading to compression if continued for long periods of time.

Pain of any type is unpleasant. If it's referred pain, it can be harder to treat and this is why it's essential you seek help to correct any problems before they get worse.

Type 2 diabetes is not a condition you must just live with. By making easy changes to your daily routine, its possible to protect your heart, kidneys, eyes and limbs from the damage often caused by diabetes, and eliminate some of the complications you may already experience. Maintaining a healthy blood sugar level means avoiding nerve damage.

What Happens in The Brain When Someone is Having an Orgasm?

The reason why each person to have sex are very diverse and complex. What happens in the brain when someone is having an orgasm?

Orgasm is a sudden movement, contraction and a wave of sexual desire. But sometimes, not everyone can achieve orgasm with the maximum. In this case, the brain plays an important role to achieve orgasm, the body sends messages to the brain.

Without the nerves that send impulses to the spinal cord and brain, orgasm is not repeated.

Similar to other areas of the body, genitals (genital organs) also contains a variety of nerve may send information to the brain to say that the feeling of being experienced. This also explains why the sensation of orgasm is different because it depends on what area is affected and the nerves involved.

All parties have a genital nerve endings which in turn is connected to a large nerve in the spinal cord.

As mentioned HowStuffWorks, Tuesday (9/3/2010) a few nerves responsible for sexual stimulation in the region, namely:

1. Hypogastric nerve stimulation transmits the functioning of the cervix in women and prostate cancer in men.

2. The stimulation of the pelvic nerves convey the role of women in the vagina and rectum in men.

3. Pudendal nerve stimulation transmits the functioning of the clitoris in women and the scrotum in men.

4. Vagus nerve stimulation transmits the functioning of the cervix, uterus and vagina.

During the existence of sexual stimulation, regions differ in the brain gets all the information and let the orgasm, and create a nice feeling.

In late 1990, scientists at the University of Groningen in the Netherlands to do research to determine brain activity during sexual stimulation.

The research team used PET to look at different regions of the brain that lights up and die during sexual activity. It was discovered that not too many differences between men and women.

"Regional brain behind the left eye, called the lateral orbitofrontal cortex during orgasm will be closed. This is a reasonable area and control behavior, so if someone has an orgasm about to lose control," said R. Jannik Georgiadis, one of the researchers.

Meanwhile, according to Dr. Gert Holstege of the brain of a person having an orgasm 95 percent of it that when people use heroin.

But there are some differences found. When a woman sexually, part of the brainstem called eriaqueductal gray (PAG) is a function of control or resist the reaction of pleasure. Also female brain also showed a decreased activity in the amygdala and hippocampus, associated with fear and anxiety.

Researchers say these differences because women need to feel safe and relaxed in sexual enjoyment. And the cortical regions associated with pain in women is activated, it shows that there is a clear relationship between pain and pleasure.

The study also shows, although women can cheat their partners reach orgasm, but his brain still show the truth.

When women were asked to simulate orgasm, brain activity in the cerebellum and other areas related to traffic control will increase. And a scan showed no brain activity similar to women who have a real orgasm.

Meanwhile, there are also people who could feel the orgasm, but not genital stimulation such as touching the nipple. Researchers believe that the feeling is sent by nipple stimulation provide the same information by stimulation of the genitals.

The Heart's Pacemaker Starts the Beat

From the SAN to the AVN and finally Purkinje fibres, all these structures play a vital part in ensuring the heart beats regularly and continually. During times of stress our heartbeat increases, during times of relaxation, our heartbeat decreases. This is caused by other chemicals in our bodies called hormones, released to either slow or quicken the SAN firing process.

The sinoatrial node (SAN) is located between the right atrium and the superior vena cava. The SAN is self-contained and does not require stimulation from the nervous system; although it is innervated by sympathetic and parasympathetic nerves, which regulate the heart beat. The SAN is the heart's electrical pacemaker. It is responsible for the intrinsic rhythmic activity of the heart. The SAN is composed of closely and densely packed pacemaker cells. The $Na+$ channels of the pacemaker cells are more open than other cardiac cells and the resting potential is less negative than the other cells. The action potential of pacemaker cells is due to voltage gated $Ca2+$ channels not the usual $Na+$ and $K+$ ions. Following a resting potential, $Na+$ ions permeate the cells more readily than $K+$ ions, making the inside more negative causing $Ca2+$ channels to open, the membrane potential rises causing an action potential to generate and start the chain reaction.

Cardiac muscle cells are in electrical contact with each other via gap junctions, enabling action potentials to spread rapidly, causing the cells to contract in unison.

As the action potential is generated in the SAN, the signals pass quickly through the electrically joined cardiac muscles of the atria, like a lit fuse, and they contract in unison, causing the right and left atria to contract.

The electrical wave continues to the junction of the atria and ventricles and stimulates the atrioventricular node (AVN). Before the AVN fires, however, there is a delay of 0.1 seconds to allow the atria to finish contracting. When the AVN does fire, the electrical impulse travels through the atrioventricular bundle or bundle of His, which are specialist larger Purkinje fibres emanating from the AVN. The His divide into finer Purkinje fibres, through which the current flows, finally across conducting fibres, ending at the apex of the myocardium of the ventricles at the base of the heart. Here the ventricular contraction begins, sweeping upwards and outwards through the ventricles, pumping blood into the pulmonary artery and aorta. The process then repeats itself, up to 76 beats/processes per minute for a normal healthy adult at rest.

Although the electrical activity within the SAN is not transmitted from the sympathetic or parasympathetic nerves, they do play a part in regulation of the heart's beat.

The sympathetic nerves originate in the vasomotor centre of the brain, situated in the medulla. They travel via the spinal cord to the sympathetic ganglion and finally to the SAN, AVN and atria/ventricle myocardium.

The parasympathetic nerves travel from the cardio inhibitory centre of the brain, in the medulla, via the 10th cranial nerve (vagus nerve), to the parasympathetic ganglion and finally to the SAN, AVN and atrial muscle.

The sympathetic and parasympathetic nerves have opposite effects on the heart's beat. The sympathetic nerves use the neurotransmitters adrenalin and noradrenalin to increase the force and rate of the heartbeat. These are the "fight, flight and fright" hormones. When we are frightened, threatened or facing other stressful situations, the release of these neurotransmitters causes the heart to beat faster. If we engage in exercise, they are released to ensure the heart beats faster to provide blood more readily to muscles.

Parasympathetic nerves use the neurotransmitter acetylcholine to decrease the force and rate of the heartbeat, for example, when we sleep, relax, the heart does not have to beat so quickly.

Therefore the SAN is continually monitored and kept in check by these sets of nerves. This process is called cholinergic vagal input or vagal restraint.

Promising Studies for Chiropractic Care and Your Heart

Each year 21 million Americans die and over 1/3 of these deaths are due to just on cause- heart disease. Everyone knows that a poor diet, lack of exercise, smoking and genetics are risk factors for cardiovascular problems.

A less familiar factor affecting heart function is the nerve system.

Nerves from the upper back (sympathetic) stimulate the heart to beat faster and more forcefully. The vagus nerve (parasympathetic) passes through the skull and down to the heart to slow the pulse and decrease the power of each contraction. Normal function is the result of a balance between these two systems. Spinal misalignments, which interfere with these nerves (vertebral subluxations), can adversely affect heart function.

A number of studies have shown great promise for patients with heart disease and blood pressure problems by correcting vertebral subluxations with chiropractic adjustments. A 1995 study found improvement in cardiac arrhythmias after neck and upper back adjustments. A 1988 study, involving 21 hypertensive patients, found a statistically significant decrease in both systolic and disstolic blood pressure in the active treatment group, but not in the placebo or control groups.

A 1993 case study of a 38 year old man with a 14 year history of hypertension dramatically shows the potential benefits of chiropractic care. The side effects of his two medications included a bloating sensation, depression, fatigue, impotence, and low back pain. After seven visits all medication was discontinued. His blood preassure was normal and all the undesirable side effect symptoms disappeared.

Chiropractic care does not attempt to treat or cure heart disease. Adjustment simply correct vertebral subluxations which interfere with normal nerve and body function. Restoring normal nerve function allows the heart and the cardiovascular system to function at their genetic potential.

Magic Touch Massage

A weekly massage may seem an indulgence, but new research suggests it can have major health benefits. Scientists are now finding that massage can reduce blood pressure, boost the immune system, dampen harmful stress hormones and raise mood-elevating brain chemicals such as serotonin. And you can't beat massage for relaxation. All these factors, "put massage in the same category with proper diet and exercise as something that helps maintain overall health". (Newsweek, April 6, 1998)

Many of the benefits stem directly from physical manipulation. Skilled hands can press lactic acid out of the muscles after exercise, easing the pains of marathon runners and triathletes. And by dispersing fluids, massage can ease the inflammation that follows sprains and other injuries (although it shouldn't be used within the first day or two). When a woman has lymph nodes removed during a mastectomy, lymphatic fluid can collect in the arm, causing swelling. Massage is the only good treatment.

The effects aren't always so straight-forward. Massage can also stimulate nerves that carry signals from the skin and muscles to the brain, triggering changes throughout the body. Massage (as opposed to light touch) stimulates the brain's vagus nerve causing the secretion of food absorption hormones, including insulin. Nerve stimulation probably explains other benefits as well.

"Every nerve cell in the body has some connection to every other nerve cell". Even brain waves are altered by massage.

Massage is not a single discipline but a family of related arts, each offering different advantages. If you're plagued by insomnia or simply need to relax, Swedish massage, with its long soothing strokes, may be all you need. But if you suffer from painful muscle spasms or need to rehabilitate an injured joint, "deep tissue" massage may be more helpful. The technique uses greater pressure to penetrate to deeper muscle groups. "Trigger-point therapy" can help relieve pain by prodding and stretching out sensitive spots that cause aches in other parts of the body. (Think of the headache you relieve by rubbing the back of the neck.) Like exercise, massage does more for you if you engage in it regularly. But even a monthly treatment can help maintain general health. "Touch is basic to survival" say Elliot Greene, past president of AMTA. That's all the excuse anyone should need to indulge!

New Depression Treatment with FDA Approval in the Next Few Days

Within the next few days, the FDA is expected to issue its final approval of vagus nerve stimulation as a treatment for chronic or recurrent depression. Also within the next few weeks, the FDA is supposed to issue a final approval of a medical breakthrough treatment for chronic or treatment-resistant depression. Final FDA approval of vagus nerve stimulation as a therapy for chronic or recurrent treatment-resistant depression to be issued in May.

A friend of mine Charles Donovan was a patient in the FDA investigational trial of vagus nerve stimulation as a treatment for chronic or recurrent treatment-resistant depression. Vagus nerve stimulation will be the mainstream treatment for chronic or treatment-resistant depression. This is an extraordinary announcement and major step for the four million Americans suffering from chronic or treatment-resistant depression towards providing an FDA-approved, informatively labeled, long-term treatment option specifically for their lifelong and life-threatening illness.

Whichever methods you choose, remember that there are many effective methods of treatment for anxiety and depression, and that patience and persistence will eventually lead you to the healthy option that is best for you. However, for a depression treatment alternative without unwanted and oft times harmful side effects, dare I say drug-free healing using simple Yoga principles and natural methods might be your best bet, it did work for me. So empower yourself to a successful depression treatment targeting its root cause with drug-free methods of healing.

Now, not to get of the subject of depression treatment, these steps, be they a fast or a healthier diet, will ensure that the body is cleaner and well we all should know by now that a cleaner body equates to a cleaner mind. If this all sounds a bit advanced, perhaps a simpler illustration of how Yoga works effectively for depression treatment may be that it exercises the motor centers of the brain, making the blood flow away from the emotional activity center; consequently one becomes more receptive to positive thoughts. Regardless of how long you have been depressed, whether you have improved to the level you want, or at what stage you are with your depression treatment, it is imperative you take the time to learn new ways of thinking, new ways of acting and new ways of feeling.

Taking an active part in your depression treatment is essential in order for you to realize success and you should seek support from a spouse or family members so that you will always be in control of your bipolar disorder or your depression. I hope that approval of this remarkable procedure gives depression sufferers the hope to continue to seek treatment for their illness. On June 15th, the FDA's Neurological Advisory Panel recommended APPROVAL of the vagus nerve stimulator as a treatment for chronic depression.

Stimulation to the left vagus nerve has been proven to favorably modulate those ares of the brain that are responsible for mood and depression. Antidepressants are used to treat chemical imbalance in the brain, but what many do not realize is that the

135

chemical imbalance is usually a symptom of depression and not the cause. By depression there is a decreased amount of neurotransmitters in parts of the central nervous system, mainly deficiency of serotonin, but also to some extend of noradrenalin, acetylcholine, dopamine or gamma-amino-butyric acid (GABA), or the nerve cells do not react properly by stimulation from neurotransmitters.

After an eight-year investigation of vagus nerve stimulation and depression, the FDA has deemed the therapy approvable with its final and binding approval decision expected within the next two weeks. One of the most important similarities is that Vagus Nerve Stimulation treatment efficacy improves over time. If natural treatment for depression is the path you want to follow, get the very best advice you can, and get yourself back on the road to good mental health.

Measurable Results for the Length of a Breath Using Yoga?

Maybe you've been wondering what kind of results you can expect from practicing a yoga breathing technique.

Well, I sure did and I ended up doing an informal study of my yoga students to find out if indeed, measurable results were possible. I'll explain the design of my study, some of the results, the benefits, and then you can try out the first technique we practiced.

The Design

In our study, we collected data from two college PE (Functional Yoga Training) classes; 63 students taking class with me twice a week for a full semester (roughly 16 weeks).

This twice a week practice was critical to achieving a measurable result!

We measured over 11 significant parameters involving strength, flexibility, lung capacity, sleep levels and the ability to relax; performing assessments at the beginning, middle and end of the semester.

The first measurement we took was the 'length of a breath'. And I'm going to share the framework of this parameter with you.

To extend breathing capacity we worked with three very specific Functional Yoga Training breathing techniques, known in yoga as 'pranayama'. Part of this practice also included using these specialized breathing techniques while working in twisting poses, to increase respiratory capacity.

Here are some of the results:

At the beginning of the semester Group I (34 students) started out with a class average of 22.6 seconds - from the beginning of the inhale to the end of the exhale - that's roughly an 11 second inhale and an 11 second exhale.

Some of the students in the group had a total breath length of only nine seconds from inhale to exhale. That's roughly a four second inhale and a five second exhale, not unusual for a person who's never been introduced to breathing techniques.

Take a moment right now, to measure your breath from the beginning of the inhale to the end of the exhale, and find out the length of your breath. Grab a stopwatch or use a count of 1 - 1000, 2 - 1000, 3 - 1000... Make of note of this for later.

By the end of the semester, practicing the Functional Yoga Training breathing techniques we learned in class; the length of a breath (class average) was 32.2 seconds! That's a 43% increase!

Combining the results from both groups, a startling 40% (25 out of 63) of these students achieved greater than a 50% increase in the length of a breath! These 25 students had an impressive breath length at the end of the semester that ranged from 22 - 60 seconds!

These results are entirely possible for you, if you're willing to practice at least twice a week. And, if you practice even more frequently, your results can surpass what we observed in the study.

So by now I'm sure you're ready to learn one of these techniques. This first one we'll cover is a building block for all the other breathing techniques we used. This is the start of acquiring a relaxed longer breath, like the students in the study and it's called an Ujayi breath.

The Technique

Ujayi Breath:

Seated comfortably

Inhale through the nose to the back of your throat

Stay with your inhale as long as comfortable

Feel and listen to the sound of your breath as it passes the throat

Exhale from the back of your throat back out through the nose

Feel and listen to the sound of your breath as it passes the throat

Try to match the length of your exhale with the length of your inhale

Repeat for five breaths

This type of breathing conserves energy and calms the nervous system by stimulating the vagus nerve while breathing. You might wonder why that's important, I'll explain:

The vagus nerve is the tenth of twelve paired cranial nerves. It is a remarkable nerve that supplies nerve fibers to the pharynx (throat), larynx (voice box), trachea (windpipe), lungs, heart, esophagus, and the intestinal tract as far as the transverse portion of the colon.

The vagus nerve also brings sensory information back to the brain from the ear, tongue, pharynx, and larynx.

Information travels through this nerve to and from your central nervous system.

Since 1997 there's been a form of therapy available for severe clinical depression, when standard drug therapy fails, known as Vagal Nerve Stimulation. A pacemaker type of device known as a pulse generator is surgically implanted into the chest wall with a wire attached to the left vagus nerve in order to send electrical signals along the vagus nerve to the mood centers in the brain.

With this therapy the hope is that these signals will improve the symptoms of depression.

Did you know you can stimulate your own Vagus nerve with Ujayi breathing by having a focus on the sound of your breath as it passes the throat?!

Try the technique again. It's listed above, and focus once again on the sound of your breath, and the feeling it creates within your body.

How do you feel now compared to before practicing the Ujayi breath?

With a calmer nervous system, your body can take in additional oxygen and metabolize it more efficiently, leading to all kinds of positive benefits, including those signals back to the brain affecting your mood centers.

With this breath you can literally calm your own nervous system. Aside from learning how to lengthen your breath, a calmer nervous system will allow you to feel more relaxed, and we all want that!

Understanding Gastroparesis

Gastroparesis refers to delayed emptying of the stomach. Normally, the stomach muscles contract to push food along, and the gastric pylorus (which is the gateway leading to the small intestine) relaxes in order for the food to pass into the duodenum (the first part of the small intestine). A major nerve known as the Vagus nerve is responsible for the control of this movement of food from the stomach through the gastrointestinal tract.

What Causes Gastroparesis?

Any condition which damages the vagus nerve can result in delayed emptying of the stomach. The most common cause of gastroparesis is diabetes mellitus. Chronic high sugar levels cause damage to blood vessels and nerves, the vagus nerve being one that is commonly affected.

Other causes of gastroparesis include:

• Damage to the vagus nerve in abdominal surgery

• Fibromyalgia

• Parkinson's disease

• Acute illness of any kind causing transient gastroparesis

• Cancer drugs affecting gastric emptying

What are the Symptoms of Gastroparesis?

Symptoms may vary in type and severity. Some are only affected when eating solid foods, high-fibre foods, fatty foods, or very large meals. Others may develop symptoms regardless of what they eat, although certain foods typically make the symptoms worse.

Commonly experienced symptoms include:

• Feeling full without eating very much

• Abdominal bloatedness

• Feeling as if food is not being digested

• Heartburn

• Nausea

• Vomiting of undigested food. This can be delayed several hours after a meal.

• Poor apetite

• Weight loss

• Pain in the upper abdomen

How is it Diagnosed?

After taking a clinical history and performing a physical examination, your doctor may order some investigations.

Blood tests: to check for diabetes, electrolyte imbalances, signs of infection as a cause of gastroparesis

Ultrasound: to rule out gallbladder disease as a cause of symptoms

Other tests: Barium meal, gastric emptying scintigraphy, breath testing, SmartPill®

How is Gastroparesis Treated?

Treatment is generally symptomatic, as gastroparesis tends to be a chronic condition. Conditions which have lead to, or which can worsen gastroparesis, also need to be addressed. For instance, diabetes will have to be well controlled, to prevent or slow down further damage to the vagus nerve.

The following medication are often used to treat the symptoms of gastroparesis:

• Metoclopramide (maxolon)

• Domperidone (motilium)

Lifestyle and Dietary Changes:

- Eat small, more frequent meals

- Avoid foods high in fat and fibre content

- Eat softer, more easily digestible foods

Language Before Music - Music Before Language?

So what if...

you saw sound?

you could hear thought?

you could smell the correct path?

What if it were all about spirals...

It's quite likely human predecessors intuitively appreciated that the world formed around spirals and responded to the perception of sound much more holistically with their body~mind connection.

Recently (early in 2009), little furry mutants in Leipzig started making slightly lower-pitched ultrasonic whistles.

This was the result of an experiment performed at the Max Planck Institute for Evolutionary Anthropology in Leipzig, Germany. Scientists ambitiously created a strain of mouse that contains the human variant of a gene, called FOXP2.

It's a gene associated with several critical tasks, including the human capacity for language.

Not surprisingly a recent comparison of those with the new gene in place showed these mice, in fact communicate differently with each other, by using slightly lower-pitched ultrasonic whistles. What's even more intriguing: the nerve cells they grow in one region of the brain show a marked level of higher complexity than those in unaltered mice.

These anthropological explorations can help us better understand what constellation of genes and cultural practices actually underpin the capacity for language in humans.

As a rehabilitative counselor - that helps restore neuro-muscular function - related to physical equilibrium, I see a robust connection of music to human movement and communication. I surmise the appreciation of rhythm found in music originated as a survival and training tool to replicate important sounds of everyday life. The role of birds as communicators to aid human and other animal survival is a well documented precedent. Birds alarm about potential threat, sing us to sleep, are linked to cross-cultural spiritual beliefs, and perhaps represent the first earthly rhythmical entertainers.

The thought that manipulation of sound originated to enhance our survival by improving coordinated movement and communication for social interaction, reproduction, teaming and averting danger is very evident in the development of our brains and neural networks.

When we measure the emotional response to music, what is primarily examined is the personification of "meaning" -- whether the person understands the "meaning" of various audible sounds. That seems, in part, to be passed on genetically (at least pre-wired), familiarly, and easily learned over the course of life.

Having a coherent, organic system that links our body to a pre-wired process in the brain (that responds to sounds and movement we experience over a lifetime) lends to this survival rationale.

Vibration, music, rhythm and even absorption of echo-location is said to be the first language that arrives in sensate form to the body. The primordial link to a burgeoning social journey that begins in the womb. To appreciate and understand this indivisible truth -- at an elemental level -- we need only explores the effect of ambient energy (energy being nature's most basic ordering pattern) in relation to its effect on prenatal infants and its affect on communal gatherings that form the basis for personal identity (in the form of rituals of solidarity).

Let's use the discovery of the world's first flute as an example.

Dug from the Hohle Fels cave, about 14 miles southwest of the city of Ulm, by archaeologist Nicholas J. Conard of University of Tubingen in Germany in 2008, the nearly complete flute implies the first humans to occupy Europe had a fairly sophisticated musical culture. The wing bone of a griffon vulture with five precisely drilled holes in it is the oldest known musical instrument (a 35,000-year-old relic of an early human society) that seems to have contributed to improved social cohesion and new forms of individual expression of communication. Most likely, this indirectly contributed to demographic expansion of modern humans to the detriment of the culturally more conservative Neanderthals.

Social cohesion goes hand in glove with the dawn of social grouping. Humans initially gathered and lived together in a size that is based on faith, trust and familiarity that "fits" intuitively with the community of human nature. In earlier times humanity had been, just like the animals, very strongly connected to the group consciousness and acted as a group to survive. This coherence naturally generated a process of what could be termed enhanced, intuitive communication. In nature, hypercommunication has been successfully applied for millions of years to organize dynamic groupings. The organized flow of a school of fish or a flock of birds on the wing proves this dramatically. Modern man knows it only on a much more subtle level as "intuition".

Yet our primal tribal form--developed based on the sort of mental personal data assistant we carry around in our heads that matches "faces to places" and allows us to name a member of our tribe even in an unfamiliar setting. This isn't an archaic process of social formation but a primordial one. Until the most recent of human history, people dwelled in groups of "tribe size" and our inclination, even today, consistently reverts us back to that comfort zone. For example, it is no accident of modern literature that the Bard has King Lear retire from the throne but retain 100 knights around him to maintain his sense and ruler of the realm persona of "kingly" community.

While personal identity formation is literally one-half of this social understanding of music and language evolution, a vital element of "comm-unity" formation is found in the group personification of sound. To develop and experience individuality we humans had to mask, or perhaps more accurately ensconce our emerging persona in musical form and expression. It thus became an imperative of social gathering (that wished to elicit and guide emotional response) that acoustics and rhythm play an integrating role. These ambient sound aspects exercise a vicarious social role that resonated a biosphere to enliven an audience and ultimately bolster the sense of community. For cross-cultural emphasis, the Renaissance Indian ritual of Astakaliya Kirtan - in which prolonged singing is accompanied by rhythmic drumming to enchant participants is exemplar.

Smelling Sound

However, movements outside of our audible range are still rhythmic, and serve us much in the same way as audible sound. We sense movement by way of our three body balance centers. These systems all relate fluid to electrical impulse via the central nervous system (brain and spinal cord), the skeletal structure, and the musculature. It is a complex systems that works as a team to provide the right output for proper body stabilization against gravitational forces. Bodily movements depend on messages to and from the control room of the brain. The brain remembers patterns of movement via rhythm not of individual muscle interactions. So even our sense of smell can tells us direction when it is unclear.

For instance, polyvagal theory, the study of the evolution of the human nervous system and the origins of brain structures, assumes more of our social behaviors and emotional disorders are biological-that is, they are "hard wired" into us-than we usually think.

The term "polyvagal" combines "poly," meaning "many," and "vagal," which refers to the longest cranial nerve set called the vagus (affectionately known as the "wanderer" nerve). To understand the theory, a deeper understanding of the vagus nerve needs to be taken into careful consideration. This nerve is a primary component of the autonomic nervous system. The nervous system that you don't control. That causes you to do things automatically, like digest your food. The vagus nerve exits the brain stem and has branches that regulate structures in the head and in several organs, including the heart and colon. The theory proposes the vagus nerve's two different branches are related to the unique ways we react to situations we perceive as safe or unsafe by properly positioning the body for flight or fight. Significantly, this nerve uniquely interacts with the only muscles in the body that are fed by cranial and spinal nerves around the neck and upper back (sterno cleido and upper trapezius). These muscles also interlace with the olfactory aspect of the limbic brain to permit us to turn our heads instinctively to sense the direction of potential danger.

So it's easily understood how we sense sound vibration and movement with our physical body, and that our body is able to carry out cognitive tasks to support multi-tasking by the brain. Using our body in this way aids a specific type of survival intelligence. Particularly as our bodies are pre-wired to recognize rhythmic patterns, with sensors in each of our joints. This enables us to communicate, think, recall, and execute cognitive tasks in part with our bodies.

What Exactly is Gastroparesis?

Gastroparesis has a few main causes. One of the main causes is diabetes, of both type 1 and also type 2. This is largely because uncontrolled glucose levels destroy the vagus nerve.The vagus nerve has the most responsibility of all your cranial nerves. This nerve that begins in the brain, goes on through your neck, through the thorax, and into the stomach. When high blood sugars destroy this function over time, it causes many problems with digestion and stomach emptying.

What you should also understand is that the vagus nerve is made of many fibers and tissues that does a lot for your body. Other than digestion, it controls many of your motor and sensory function. When blood vessels become seriously impaired from either type of diabetes, this stomach problem is a likely problem.

A lot of vomiting such as from bulimia, anorexia, cancer drugs, and severe acid reflux disease can greatly cause a disturbance within the digestive tract itself, and over time, causes what is known as a motility problem. What is motility? Motility is defined as a spontaneous movement of a muscle. And in this case, we are speaking of stomach muscles. When this factor within the body is disturbed within the nerves to our digestive tract, many problems will manifest themselves.

Symptoms of Gastroparesis

Acid reflux is a common problem with this medical condition.

Feeling full even several hours after eating.

Constipation since the stomach fails to process food or digest much of it.

Vomiting is another dominant symptom as well. Since the vagus nerve fails to tell the stomach to digest food for whatever medical reason, you'll vomit food consumed from days before.

Diagnosing Gastroparesis

To diagnose this stomach problem, you may be given a meal that contains substances which are radioactive. Doctors will view your stomach after the meal several times to see how the meal is digesting or not. Other ways to diagnose the problem are by performing an endoscopy and also an ultrasound. Some doctors may have you swallow a special pill which is radioactive. The pill tracks what is going on inside the stomach and leaves the body in a couple days through stool. The doctor then reads the collected data of the stomach on a computer.

Treatments for Gastroparesis

It is often required to make changes to your diet in order to control this medical problem. You will have to eat foods that are easiest to digest, and avoid those foods that are harder on the stomach. Foods that have a lot of fat or fiber are not easy to digest for example, and you will probably have to avoid many of these foods. Medications can be given such as Reglan or Compazine. These help the stomach muscles move so that your stomach can empty properly.

Another radical treatment is through something called gastric electrical stimulation. This is surgical procedure where they place a device that is operated by a battery, and it sends the signals out through your body to help control the vomiting and nauseated feeling you have in severe cases. Sometimes there are people with this medical condition that will need a feeding tube in order to receive nourishment to the body. This is only done in the most severe of cases.

High Blood Pressure and Chiropractic

Raise your hand if you know someone taking drugs to lower their blood pressure. Well. That's about 100%. We ALL know someone doing that. And, I guess we all know why. "Unresolved" chronic high blood pressure can supposedly cause stroke, congestive heart failure and kidney failure. In other words, modern Medicine must coerce people through fear to take drugs to control a body function.

Unfortunately, those prescribing drugs for high blood pressure rarely know what is causing a patient's problem. In fact, they may not even stop to think that there may be a GOOD reason for a person's elevated blood pressure. It just might be that there is some condition causing their body to NEED more blood. Most prescriptions for blood pressure medications rarely consider the CAUSE of the problem, whatsoever.

Virtually all prescriptions for blood pressure drugs come in one of four categories: diuretics, beta-blockers, ACE inhibitors and calcium channel blockers. And remember, these drugs only mask the symptom of some unknown condition while having NO healing properties AND even the least toxic ones can have deadly side effects.

You might be asking "What the heck does chiropractic have to do with high blood pressure?" I'm glad you asked. While some folks think chiropractic maybe great for back pain, they rarely consider that what chiropractic adjustments really do is take pressure off either specific nerve roots or off the entire nerve system altogether, or both. For our purposes here, I want you to consider something called the Vagus Nerve.

The Vagus Nerve is a very special nerve located in an area called the brain stem. The brain stem is located just below the brain and just above the spinal cord. One of its jobs is to regulate your heart rate, blood pressure, digestion and many other functions. In fact, the Vagus Nerve is kind of like the reset switch on your computer. When things lock up, one of the first things you try is the reset button. Most times, that resolves the problem.

Everyone's heard of the body's "fight or flight" mechanism where you gear up for a fight or an to escape a life threatening situation. In our rushed and harried world, many of us stay in this "fight or flight" mode due to chronic stress. Over time, this causes chronic high blood pressure. Our diet and lack of exercise also contribute to the problem. Yet, few doctors recommend stress reduction, diet and exercise as a means of dealing with high blood pressure.

So, how do chiropractic adjustments help lower blood pressure? Specific adjustments of the bone at the top of the neck, called the

Atlas, can help reduce stress on the brain stem. Reducing stress on the brain stem can stimulate the Vagus Nerve, helping to slow down your heart rate and lower the blood pressure. There are lots of technical explanations for this. But, this book is directed at people who want to get off drugs and lower the blood pressure naturally, not someone looking to justify the use of drugs. In short, chiropractic adjustments of the upper cervical spine stimulate what's called the parasympathetic nervous system, or the reset button for the "fight or flight" mechanism.

While any good chiropractor can adjust the upper cervical spine, I believe the best results come from specific upper cervical adjustments. And you just might realize other benefits from upper cervical chiropractic adjustments, like better sleep, digestion and elimination. maybe even better sex. But, that's a topic for another day.

Can High-Pitched Sounds Be a Cure for Tinnitus?

Research workers could possibly have formulated a cure for tinnitus, the prolonged ringing in the ears which harms the day-to-day lives of tens of thousands of People all over the world. During medical tests, research workers made it possible to cease the aggravating sound disturbance simply by stirring a certain nerve within the neck whilst using some sort of high-pitched tone directly towards the ears. This particular technique which refreshes the brain have been subjected to testing in rats with a huge success. Scientific tests upon human beings are expected to start off in the succeeding couple of months.

Close to one in ten, about ten percent, grown ups in the United Kingdom are affected with irreversible tinnitus and about 600,000 already possess it horribly enough to have an effect on their standard of living.

This condition can easily have an affect on either ear and is particularly referred to as a ringing noise, even though it could likewise take the kind of high-pitched wails, rattling, rushing sound or a low-toned beep. The ringing in the ears can often be brought about by being exposed to over the top noise, which in turn damages the cells inside the inner ear that broadcast sound information towards the human brain.

Research workers are convinced that the human brain attempts to make amends for the omitted signals, resulting to what is referred to as phantom sounds. Some other reasons behind the ringing in the ears involve injuries and also the normal process of aging. American research workers conducted studies on the topic of "rats with tinnitus" intended to result in alterations in the auditory cortex, which is the section of the brain which reacts to sound.

By means of stimulating the vagus nerve, a sizable nerve going from your neck and head towards the abdominal area, electrically by using a tiny electrode while also playing some high-pitched sound, these people were able to remove the ringing of the ears on the test subjects.

Remedied test subjects demonstrated reactions that pointed out that the tinnitus had ceased the journal Nature described. Those animals which failed to take advantage of the therapy carried on to produce the signs and symptoms of tinnitus.

Research head Dr Michael Kilgard, from the University of Texas in Dallas, mentioned that the secret is that, in contrast to earlier solutions, they were not covering up tinnitus. He and his group were retuning the brain originating from a condition in which it produces ringing in the ears towards a condition which doesn't produce the ringing in the ears. They were getting rid of the origin of the ringing in the ears. Once the vagus nerve is aroused it emits chemical substances that may modify brain connectivity. Individuals getting involved in the human test in Europe is going to go through vagus nerve arousal combined with sounds at every day treatment periods for a number of weeks.

The particular stimulation is going to be sent using a wireless electrode surgically connected to the vagus nerve on the left.

How the Mind Can Become your Best Healer?

Did you know that your brain actually has the power to heal you? No! Then you must know that according to scientists the brain has the ability to stimulate our immune system for fighting and combating diseases.

Dr. Kevin Tracey, an immunologist, neurosurgeon and the director of the Feinstein Institute of Medical Research in New York, first came up with this fantastic scientific discovery. The finding required two decades of careful experiments on Dr. Tracey's part. The influence behind his finding - a little girl all of 11 months, named Janice, who had suffered 75 percent burns from boiling water all over her body. She developed severe sepsis, which is a condition that has the immune system overreacting to a bacterial function.

Severe sepsis

The little girl could not be saved, and this unfortunate incident compelled Dr. Tracey to investigate the cause of severe sepsis. He discovered that the stimulation of the vagus nerve, which runs from the human brainstem to the belly and regulates our breathing, heartbeat and intestines has the capacity to stop severe sepsis.

Now how does it do so? The vagus nerve stops severe sepsis by making use of the neurochemicals for activating the immune cells. This prevents the release of the alarm molecules, that cause spur inflammation and damage. Dr. Tracey found a brain circuit that could make the vagus nerve switch off the inflammation. Thus, a connection between the brain and immune system was found, which according to Dr. Tracey was the 'inflammatory reflex'.

Wonders of the brain

Normally during inflammation, the brain helps the immune system to heal it, but in severe sepsis the reflex fails. So, the solution is to intake drugs for activating the reflex and bringing about a reduction in the chronic low-grade inflammation.

You can also try meditation for thwarting diseases. You can even control your brain to combat disease and calm inflammation, by slowing the heartbeat to modify the vagus nerve activity. This also slows down the spreading rate of some cancers.

A reduction in stress through meditation can fight cancer. Norepinephrine, the stress hormone can make the lab-grown cancer cells release two compounds, which helps them move through the body and spread. Another compound released will encourage tumor growth with nutrients. So, reduce your stress levels, the key to better living is in your hands.

Out of The Box Thinking for Insanely Fast and Easy Weight Loss

If you are like most people, you are probably using exercise methods out of a magazine or from your trainer. The truth is that these are ordinary and old methods that will only get you ordinary results. You can not expect to be ahead of the rest of the pack doing the same things as everyone else does. This will get you nowhere fast.

There are only a few who are at the top of the game. These people do things "outside of the box". They think differently than everyone else and their results show. They get fast results and the results are effective.

So here is what you need to know that will change the way you think, so you can develop the new attitude of intrigue and enthusiasm, and go into your exercises with this attitude, because 80% of it is attitude.

Look at your body from a biological perspective. How does your body burn fat and use energy?

In order for this to take place cells need to be phosphorylized. Signalling takes place in your cells and this signalling sets off a cascade of reactions in cells to use energy and burn fat. So how do we increase signalling?

There are various supplements you can take that increase cell signalling and allow for greater cellular energy utilisation.

Some of these supplements include: ALCAR(acetyl-l-carnitine), Leucine, isoleucine, creatine. These bodybuilding supplements are some of the most effective ways to burn fat and increase energy burning.

A lot of people use these things, but have little idea of the actual science behind them. It is important to know what they actually do, so you can have the right attitude about exercise.

When I say that 80% of your weight loss efforts are attitude, this is the truth. The majority of people go into their workouts lost and have no clue what is happening at a cellular level.

It`s like trying to do something for the first time you have no idea about. Knowledge provides intrigue and enthusiasm and this is fuel for amazing results!

Another "outside the box" thought is the mechanism that controls/regulates your gut. The vagus nerve is the medium which allows the brain and gut to connect to each other. Through deep breathing and relaxation you are able to activate the vagus nerve.

So, think about it...The more deep breathing you do the more effective you become at activating the vagus nerve and having conscious control over your gut.

The more the vagus nerve is active, the more you will be able to send oxygen and activity to that part of the body.

The key principle I am trying to lay out here is that with regular practice you will greatly enhance your control in your abdomen area and boost your fat burning, muscle building ability!

Think about these ideas and allow yourself to become intrigued by the thought of totally different ways to lose weight and reach your fitness goals. You will be trying something different than everyone else, so that alone gives you an edge!

Vagus Nerve Stimulation Approaches

The vagus nerve does not have to be shocked to sculpt. It may likewise be toned and augmented like some muscles. Here are some simple things you can do that may improve your wellbeing markedly:

1. Positive Social Relationships -- A research had participants believe compassionately about the others while quietly replicating positive phrases about family and friends. When compared with the controls, the meditators demonstrated a general growth in positive feelings such as calmness, happiness, and expectation after finishing the course. These positive ideas of others resulted in an advancement in vagal nerve function noticed in heart-rate variability. The results also revealed a slimmer vagus nerve compared to when only meditating.

2. Cold -- "Cold vulnerability, for example cold showers stimulates the nerve too," states Mentore.

Studies indicate that if your body adjusts to cold, your fight or flight (perceptible) system decreases as well as your break and digest (parasympathetic) method raises --and that is evidenced by the vagus nerve. Any sort of intense cold exposure such as drinking ice cold water may boost vagus nerve stimulation.

3. Gargling -- Another home remedy to get the under-stimulated vagus nerve would be to gargle water. Gargling really stimulates the muscles of the pallet that are fired from the vagus nerve.

4. Singing And Chanting -- Humming, mantra chanting, hymn singing, also optimistic lively singing all raise heart rate variability (HRV) in somewhat different manners. Basically, singing is similar to triggering a vagal pump delivering out waves that are relaxing. Singing at the top of your lungs causes the muscles at the rear of the neck to trigger the vagus. Singing in unison, which is frequently performed in churches and synagogues, additionally raises HRV and vagus function. Singing was proven to boost oxytocin, also called the love hormone since it makes people feel closer to one another.

5. Massage -- It's possible to excite your vagus nerve by massaging your toes as well as your neck across the carotid sinus, located across the carotid arteries on each side of your throat. A throat massage can help reduce seizures. A foot massage can decrease your pulse and blood pressure. An anxiety massage may also trigger the vagus nerve. These massages are utilised to assist babies in gaining fat

by stimulating gut features, chiefly mediated by triggering the vagus nerve.

6. Laughter -- Happiness along with laughter are all normal immune boosters. Laughter stimulates the vagus nerve-stimulation. Research demonstrates how laughter raises HRV in a group atmosphere.

There are many case reports of people experiencing from bliss and this might due to the vagus nerve/parasympathetic method being aroused a lot of. Fainting may come after bliss in addition to coughing, itching, swallowing or gut movement--most of which can be aided along by vagus activation.

7. Yoga And Tai Chi -- Both raise vagus nerve action along with your lymphatic system generally. Various studies have revealed that yoga increases GABA, a calming neurotransmitter on your brain. Researchers think it does so by "stimulating vagal afferents (fibers)," which boost activity in the nervous system. This is particularly valuable for people who struggle with depression or anxiety.

Research reveals that tai chi can also 'improve vagal modulation.'

8. Breathing Deeply And Gradually -- Your heart and throat contain neurons which have receptors called baroreceptors, which control blood pressure and also transmit the adrenal signal to your brain. This triggers your vagus nerve which connects to your heart to reduce blood pressure and heart rate. Slow breathing, using a roughly equivalent quantity of time of breathing out and in, raises the sensitivity of baroreceptors and vagal activation. Breathing about 5-6 breaths per second by a normal adult can be quite valuable.

9. Exercise -- Exercise raises the brain's growth hormone, which supports your brain's mitochondria, and also aids in reversing cognitive decline. Nonetheless, it's been demonstrated to excite the vagus nerve, which contributes to beneficial brain and psychological health consequences. Mild exercise stimulates gut circulation, which can be due to the vagus nerve.

10.   Coffee Enemas -- Enemas are similar to sprints to the vagus nerve. Increasing the gut increases vagus nerve stimulation, which can be done with enemas. This cleanse is achieved by increasing the liver's ability to neutralize toxins from the bloodstream and transmitting them into the bile.

In the procedure, the liver cleans itself since it releases the poisonous bile to the small, then large intestine for evacuation. The whole blood supply circulates through the liver every 3 minutes. By keeping the java 12 to 15 minutes, the blood vessels tend to clot a few days for cleanup, like a dialysis therapy. The water content from this java stimulates intestinal peristalsis and aids in empting the large intestine together with the collected toxic bile.

11. Nervana -- This wearable merchandise transmits a gentle electric wave through the left ear canal to stimulate the body's vagus nerve, whereas still syncing it with hearing, which subsequently stimulates the release of endorphins in the brain which causes a relaxing feeling throughout your system.

12. Relax -- Learning how to be calm could possibly be the No. 1 factor to keep your vagus nerve stimulation toned. Based on Hoffman, many relaxing actions will stimulate the vagus nerve.

Vagus Nerve Exercises

- Utilizing Breathing to Decrease Pain

You can learn how to work with breathing exercises to shift your attention away from annoyance. The human brain processes one particular thing at one time. If you concentrate on the rhythm of your breathing, then you are not concentrated on the annoyance.

The minute we expect pain, the majority of us often atop breathing and hold our breath.

Breath holding triggers the fight/flight/freeze reaction, it is inclined to raise the feeling of stiffness, pain, nervousness, or anxiety. It is possible to go as follows: Take a deep breath in your stomach (i.e. extending your diaphragm) for the count of five, then pause, then exhale slowly through a little hole into your mouth. While resting most men and women take roughly 10 to 14 breaths per minute. To enter parasympathetic/ comfort / recovery mode it's best to lower your breath to 7 breaths a minute. Exhaling throughout your mouth rather than nose makes your breathing a conscious process, and can help you to detect your breath easily.

As you decrease your breaths each minute and enter parasympathetic manner, your muscles will relax, decreasing your anxieties and worries. The oxygen supply to the body's cells raises and this aids in creating endorphins, your body's feel-good hormones. Tibetan monks practice 'mindful breathing' for a long time, but there's not anything mysterious about it. It is possible to improve your experience by imagining you inhale IN joy, and exhale OUT gratitude. These early techniques will also improve memory, combat depression, reduce blood pressure, or heartbeat, and also enhance your immune system -- and it is totally free!

- 'OM' Chanting

A fascinating study was conducted from the International Journal Of Yoga at 2011, in which 'OM' chanting was contrasted with pronunciation of 'SSS,' also as a break condition to find out whether chanting is more stimulatory to the vagus nerve. The analysis found the chanting really was more powerful than the 'sss' pronunciation and also even the rest condition. Successful 'OM' chanting is connected with the encounter of a tingling feeling around the ears and also across the entire body. It's expected that this sort of feeling can also be transmitted via the auricular branch of the vagus nerve and also can create limbic (HPA axis) deactivation.

The way to chant?
Hold on the vowel (o) section of this 'OM' for 5 minutes, then continue to the consonant (m) component for another 10 seconds. Keep on chanting for 10 minutes. Conclude with a few deep breaths and finish with gratitude.

- Cold Water

Physical exercise induces an increase in sympathetic activity (HPA axis - fight/flight, anxiety reaction), together with cerebral withdrawal (resting, digesting, recovery (immune system), leading to high heart rates (HR). Studies have discovered that cold water facial immersion is apparently a straightforward and effective way of instantly hastening post-exercise parasympathetic reactivation through the vagus nerve, and sparking a decrease in heart rate, motility of the intestines, and it also works to strengthen the immune system. It's also powerful in an non-exercise surrounding to trigger the vagus nerve. During cold-water head immersion people stayed seated and flexed their head into a bowl of cold water. The facial skin is immersed so the brow, eyes, and also two-thirds of the lips were underwater. Water temperature was kept at 10-12°C.

- Increased Salivation

The calmer the brain and also the deeper the comfort, the simpler the stimulation of salivation is. The mouth can create copious amounts of spit, you are aware that the Vagus Nerve was aroused and the body is in the concentric mode. To stimulate salivation, attempt relaxing and relax in a chair and envision a hot lemon.

Since your mouth fills with saliva, then simply put your tongue within this tub (if this does not occur, simply fill your mouth with a small number of warm water and then put your tongue out within the bathroom. Only the custom of relaxing will trigger the secretion of saliva).

Now unwind farther, and feel that your hands, toes, buttocks, and back of the throat and head are all calming. Breathe deeply in this setting and remain here as long as possible.

Vagus nerve stimulation (VNS) has been demonstrated to have numerous health advantages. As an instance, researchers in Boston University School of Medicine (BUSM), New York Medical College, along with the Columbia College of Physicians and Surgeons examined evidence that demonstrates that yoga could possibly be successful in treating patients using behavioral emotional and health care conditions, such as depression, stress, high blood pressure and coronary artery disease.

The way they think it works is that anxiety causes an imbalance in the autonomic nervous system, in addition to under-activity of both gamma amino-butyric acid (GABA), an inhibitory neurotransmitter. Low GABA levels happen in stress disorders, post-traumatic anxiety disease, depression, epilepsy and chronic pain. Researchers discovered that stimulating the vagus nerve increases GABA levels and may explain why VNS functions to reduce seizure frequency, in addition to the indications of depression.

Earlier research performed by BSMU Researchers revealed that people who did yoga improved their GABA levels while diminishing symptoms of stress, whereas research participants who had been part of their walking group demonstrated no increase in GABA levels. Another study performed with patients having chronic low-back pain revealed the group who did yoga intervention reacted with greater GABA levels along with a substantial decrease in pain compared to those who received only standard care.

- 3-D Breath Breakdown

Shift heart rate variability and Increase vagal tone with what Hitzmann requires for the 3-D Breath Breakdown. (detailed directions about the best way best to conduct this breath arrangement are available here). "That is so easy to perform," Alter says. "It directly raises heart-rate variability and enables an individual to control an integral element of their autonomic nervous system by means of this clever diaphragmatic procedure. By slowing down and focusing on the path of the diaphragmatic movement, you change the method by which in which the brainstem indicates that the diaphragm contracts because it does it 25,000 times every day once you breathe and do not think about doing it."

- 50-second Facelift

"The jaw is related to the two Trigeminal and vagus nerve-stimulation," describes Hitzmann," and frequently misalignment of the chin may lead to reduced vagal tone. If you've had dentures or a lot of mouth function, or possess unstable buttocks and inadequate foot integrity and strength, you're at risk for reduced vagal tone.

By stimulating the veins in which the vagus nerve cells sits outside from the ears, then it is possible to reduce the compression that the tissue frequently has in the bottom of the skull. This is often a culprit of vagal problems missed in therapy. Sometimes the nerve is really good, however the tissues surrounding it induces imbalances in its own link in the head to gut. By discharging the cells within this field together with the 50-second Facelift method, it's possible to quickly raise the equilibrium and linking the vagus nerve should work effectively."

- Gentle Inversions

"Move upside (ish) to awaken," says Miller. "Educating yourself to ensure your muscles and center are somewhat higher than your brain. Excites the strain detectors --that the baroreceptors-- around the face of the neck inside the carotid arteries. They relay messages right to the vagus nerve, which reacts by constricting all of the blood vessels and slowing the breath speed. The final result? It slows down controlling output and accelerates parasympathetic dominance."

- Supra-Clavicle Release (aka Neck Gnar)

"Your rectal anterior neck is loaded with stress points wherever your vagus nerve can be massaged," explains Miller. "You do not need a great deal of stress to trigger the relaxation response. Try out the status technique to massage to the scalenes which overlay your own vagus and believe your entire day will become fresh."

Breathing methods and specific lifestyle habits which include breathing exercises, such as meditation and yoga, are all fantastic methods to stimulate the vagus nerve obviously," says Ilan Danan, MD, neurologist in the Kerlan-Jobe Center for Sports Neurology and Pain Medicine in Kerlan-Jobe Orthopaedic Clinic in Los Angeles, Calif. "Other items that people do every day, whether they are aware of it or not, act to stimulate the vagus nerve-stimulation, too. Including functions, like singing or laughing, which then act to improve heart rate variability, leading to vagus nerve stimulation."

Recommended Meals

Digestion along with the Vagus Nerve

The vagus nerve is part of the sysytem which informs the gut to put out amino juices and acids, and also to begin the motions of the intestine. As soon as we chew our food we initiate the practice of blending the fibers within our meals with the amino enzymes and acids which start to break down food, until it reaches the gut, before flowing to the small and then large intestine.

If the vagus nerve is not getting or sending the right signals, the stream of food-mixed-with-acid throughout the intestine is slowed. This usually means that overgrowths of yeast, bacteria or parasites -- also as consumed toxins and hormones the body tries to remove from your system -- are going through the intestine at a lesser pace. IBS and SIBO threat are raised with increased exposure to germs, waste products, possibly worsening any diseases present. Exposure to more hormones than the human body had intended on may throw hormones out of balance (discussed further below).

Vagus Nerve, both MMC along with SIBO

In the case of Small Intestine Bacterial Overgrowth (SIBO) the migrating motor complex (MMC) from the intestine isn't behaving optimally.

I love to consider MMC as the caboose of a tiny train going through our bowels. You eat, along with the consumed food, together with amino enzymes and acids, is packed on a vehicle on the rail, to be transferred by means of your entire body and outside like a blossom. Every single time you eat, the train must stop and return to the peak of the paths to pick up food.

A couple of things can halt the train. Reduced vagus nerve shooting is a significant contributor to both MMC dysregulation. Psychotherapy is just another one for certain. The train must proceed all of the way via Central Station, the location right after your gut (the duodenum) into the final stop downtown, the anus.

This should be a one-time excursion, and the train must leave the channel and reach the end of the street every 90-120 minutes. Each time you bite, the train must stop and return to pick this up a fresh food-passenger, slowing down the movement of food through your digestive tract, which may result in bacterial overgrowth and enhanced toxin intake within the torso.

The MMC may be get derailed or perplexed by injury, anxiety, and other lifestyle variables, to be discussed in depth in additional posts.

178

#Low Stomach Acid

People with IBS, heartburn, nausea as well as other digestive problems frequently have low stomach acidity, which also can be quite a vagus nerve problem. The vagus nerve arouses the cells from the gut to release histamine, which assists the body to distribute the stomach acid that you need to break down your food.

11 Tactics To Reduce Vagus Nerve Work For Improved Gut & Mental Health

1. Try deep breathing or meditation (or even both!) .

Deep breathing is among the very simple yet powerful tactics to stimulate the vagus nerve. Whenever your brain is a couple of counts more than your inhale, then the vagus nerve sends a signal to your brain to turn on your nervous system. Try this workout: Sit for 2 seconds in, and then four seconds outside, using a 1 count pause near the peak of the inhale plus a 1 count pause at the base of the exhale. Numerous studies also encourage the ability of meditation to enhance sleep, pain, hunger, stress, and digestive function using an immediate impact upon vagal tone.

2. Go to a yoga course.

Engaging in regular mild exercise like yoga increases gastric motility— the contractions of the adrenal muscle are essential for the movement of food through the gastrointestinal tract--so it does so through stimulating the vagus nerve.

3. Simply take a cold shower.

Look at finishing your bathing with a one-minute burst of chilly water, and do not be scared to go out for a walk if it is chilly. Studies indicate that intense cold exposure triggers the vagus nerve-stimulation, in addition to different neurons around the vagus nerve pathway, also resulting in a change toward autonomic nervous system action.

4. Eat foods full of tryptophan.

Dietary Tryptophan is metabolized in the intestine and might assist the astrocytes--cells in the brain and spinal cord control inflammation, which might enhance communication From the gut into the brain through the vagal messenger walkway. These meals include spinach, seeds, peas, and poultry.

5. Keep a wholesome weight.

Gut and stomach inflammation may disrupt vagal action and negatively alter the link between the brain and the GI tract. Therefore, if you are obese, your very best choice is to embrace sustainable practices which will cause long-term weight reduction. My information: Move your system every day and concentrate on consuming a diet high in many different fruits and vegetables, together with seeds, nuts, and legumes like the Mediterranean diet.

6. Ensure that you poop every day.

Eat loads of fiber-rich foods daily (target for 25-plus g), and keep regular sleep routines to enable your body to move to a daily rhythm. Healthful removal of waste ensures significantly less stagnation of inflammatory foods residues from the colon, and also a much less hospitable environment for undesirable organisms which could impair communication between the gut and brain.

7. Nix sugar in your diet plan.

Excessive sugar causes chronic inflammation but also soothes cell feedback loops along with other signaling pathways, and also inflammation of the GI tract disease lining allows germs to perpetuate inflammatory signals into the brain.

8. Pop a probiotic.

Along with bettering your ingestion of sugar to boost a wholesome gut and keep optimum gut-brain signaling, look at adding fermented foods along with a probiotic to a daily diet. Research proves that gut bacteria can in fact trigger the vagus nerve. In 1 study, mice which were given the probiotic Lactobacillus rhamnosus experienced improved GABA creation and a decrease in anxiety, depression, and stress. But this favorable effect didn't happen among mice whose vagus nerve was eliminated.

9. Should you consume plenty of creature protein, scale.

Red eggs and meat include choline, which may be helpful for you, but if consumed in excess will be switched into trimethylamine N-oxide (TMAO), a chemical that's been related to cardiovascular and inflammation troubles. Decreased consumption of those foods can reduce inflammation and permit the vagus nerve to regulate cerebral and sympathetic vitals like blood pressure and heartbeat.

10. Contemplate intermittent fasting.

Some research suggests that fasting and dietary restriction may trigger the vagus nerve. And provided that fasting's host of additional advantages --from enhanced cognitive functioning for weight loss to decreased inflammation it could possibly be well worth a try. The very best part: The fasting window does not have to be that much time to reap several fantastic advantages.

11. Belt out your favorite song.

Research also shows that singing includes a biologically calming effect, that has all to do with all the vagus nerve. Go ahead, sing with the radio if you are in the car --or even better, when you're taking a cold shower!

Broad Autonomic Effects

One important drug that affects the immune system generally isn't a pharmaceutical curative agent connected with the system. This drug is nicotine in smoking. The effects of smoking in the nervous system are very significant in thinking about the function smoking may play in wellness.

All of ganglionic neurons of this autonomic procedure, at the sympathetic and parasympathetic ganglia, are triggered by ACh released from preganglionic fibers. Even the ACh receptors on these neurons have the nicotinic kind, meaning they are ligand-gated ion stations. After the neurotransmitter released from the preganglionic fiber binds to the receptor protein, then a station opens to permit positive ions to cross the cell membrane. The outcome is depolarization of the ganglia. Nicotine serves as an ACh analog in these synapses, therefore whenever someone takes from the medication, it complies with those ACh receptors and triggers the ganglionic neurons, making them depolarize.

Ganglia of both branches are activated equally from this drug. For most target organs within your system, this leads to no net change. The rival inputs into the machine cancel out each other and nothing important happens. By way of instance, the sympathetic system may cause sphincters in the digestive tract to contract, restricting digestive propulsion, but also the neural system may cause the contraction of other organs in the gastrointestinal tract, and this will attempt to induce the contents of their digestive tract combined. The final result is that the food really doesn't move along and the digestive tract hasn't substantially changed.

Allergic Impact

The neurochemistry of this sympathetic system relies upon the adrenergic system. Norepinephrine and epinephrine influence goal effectors by binding into the α-adrenergic or β-adrenergic receptors. Medicines which influence the sympathetic system impact these compound systems.

The medication can be categorized by whether they improve the purposes of the operating system or disrupt those purposes. A medication that enhances adrenergic role is called a sympathomimetic medication, whereas a medication that interrupts adrenergic purpose is a sympatholytic medication.

Sympathomimetic Drugs

If the sympathetic system isn't Functioning properly or the entire body is in a condition of homeostatic imbalance, so all these medications act at postganglionic terminals and synapses from the sympathetic efferent pathway. These medications either bind to certain adrenergic receptors and mimic norepinephrine in the synapses between sympathetic postganglionic fibers along with their aims, or they raise the creation and release of norepinephrine from postganglionic fibers. Additionally, to boost the potency of adrenergic compounds discharged from the fibers, a few of the drugs can block the elimination or reuptake of the neurotransmitter in the synapse.

An average sympathomimetic medication is Phenylephrine, that can be a frequent ingredient in decongestants. It may likewise be used to enhance the pupils and also to increase blood pressure. Phenylephrine is called a α1-adrenergic agonist, which means that it evolves into a particular adrenergic receptor, sparking an answer. Within this function, phenylephrine will seep into the adrenergic receptors at bronchioles in the lungs and make them dilate. By launching these constructions, accumulated mucus could be removed from the lower respiratory tract.

Sympatholytic Drugs

Drugs which interfere with sympathetic role are known as sympatholytic, or sympathoplegic, medications. They mostly function as an antagonist into the adrenergic receptors. They obstruct the capacity of norepinephrine or epinephrine to bind to the receptors so the result is "cut" or even "requires a blow off," to reference the endings"-lytic" and also"-plegic," respectively. The different drugs of the course will be particular to α-adrenergic or even β-adrenergic receptors, or into their own receptor subtypes.

Probably the most recognizable sort of sympatholytic drug would be the β-blockers. These medications are usually used to treat coronary disease since they obstruct the β-receptors related to vasoconstriction and cardio acceleration. By enabling blood vessels to dilate, or maintaining heart rate from growing, these medications may enhance cardiac function at a compromised system, like for an individual who has congestive heart failure or that has endured a heart attack.

A few common variations of β-blockers are all metoprolol, which specifically blocks the β2-receptor, also propranolol, which nonspecifically cubes β-receptors. There are several other medications which are α-blockers and may impact the sympathetic system in an identical manner.

Other applications for sympatholytic drugs Are as antianxiety drugs. An example of this can be clonidine, that can be an α-agonist. The sympathetic system is connected with stress about the point which the sympathetic answer could be known as "combat, flight, or even fright." Clonidine can be used for different therapies besides hypertension and stress, such as pain ailments and attention deficit hyperactivity disorder.

Parasympathetic Consequences

Medicines affecting parasympathetic functions may be categorized into the ones that increase or diminish action at postganglionic terminals. Parasympathetic postganglionic fibers discharge ACh, along with the receptors on your goals are muscarinic receptors. There are lots of sorts of muscarinic receptors, M1--M5, however, the drugs aren't typically unique to the particular kinds.

Parasympathetic drugs may be muscarinic agonists or antagonists or have side consequences on the cholinergic system. Drugs that improve cholinergic effects are known as parasympathomimetic drugs, whereas people who inhibit cholinergic effects are also known as anticholinergic medications.

Pilocarpine is a nonspecific muscarinic agonist commonly utilized as a treatment for ailments of the eye. It reverses mydriasis, for example is brought on by phenylephrine, also may be administered following an eye examination.

Together with constricting the pupil during the smooth muscle of the iris, pilocarpine may also bring about the ciliary muscle to deal with. This may start perforations at the bottom of the retina, which allows to the drainage of aqueous humor in the anterior compartment of the eye and, thus, reducing esophageal pressure linked to atherosclerosis.

Atropine and scopolamine are part of a category of muscarinic antagonists which include the Atropa genus of crops which have belladonna or deadly nightshade (Figure 3). The title of these crops, belladonna, describes how extracts from this plant have been used for dilating the pupil. The active compounds from using this plant block the muscarinic receptors in the iris and permit the pupil to dilate, which is deemed appealing since it makes the eyes look bigger.

Individuals are automatically drawn to anything with bigger eyes, which stems in how the proportion of eye-to-head dimensions differs in babies (or infant animals) and may evoke an emotional reaction. The attractive use of belladonna infusion was basically acting with this particular response. Atropine is no more utilized within this decorative capacity for motives linked to another title for the plant, and this can be deadly nightshade. Suppression of neurological function, particularly when it will become systemic, may be deadly. Autonomic regulation is interrupted and anticholinergic symptoms grow. The berries of the plant are highly poisonous, but may be confused for different berries. The antidote for atropine or scopolamine poisoning is pilocarpine.

CONCLUSION

The vagus nerve, is the longest cranial nerve in the body, innervates the abdominal and cervical organs, including the autonomic, cardiovascular, respiratory, gastrointestinal, immune, and endocrine systems. The vagus nerve is an integral part of this autonomic nervous system (ANS) comprising 80 percent afferent and 20 percent efferent nerve fibers. Even the vagal afferent fibers feel an array of stimuli, such as stress, fever, compounds, osmotic stress, and swelling. These sensory signs are accumulated in the vagal nuclei and therefore are sent to multiple brain areas. After being processed in the brain, regulatory signs are transmitted from the vagal efferent fibers.

Vagal efferent fibers, which arise in the nucleus ambiguous and the dorsal motor nucleus, are mainly cholinergic, with acetylcholine (ACh) as their important neurotransmitter. Imbalances at the ANS, that can be characterized by a decrease in vagal tone accompanied by enhanced sympathetic activity, are related to disease development and negative clinical consequences, tripping many cardiovascular diseases, like heart failure, arrhythmia and hypertension.

Lots of studies have revealed that increased vagal action reduces cardiovascular risk variables in both animal models and patients. However, the functions of medication that trigger vagal nerves